Blood Group Antigens and Antibodies

Marjory Stroup, M.T. (ASCP) SBB
Director, Technical Resources
Immunodiagnostics

Margaret Treacy
Manager, Technical Literature
Immunodiagnostics

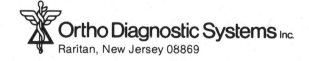 Ortho Diagnostic Systems Inc.
Raritan, New Jersey 08869

Preface

This book is intended to aid those who teach medical technology students, entry level blood bank technologists and clinical pathology residents. It reflects our philosophy of teaching which is to emphasize concepts. We believe the learner who masters the concepts of immunohematology will be able to judge the significance of test results rather than simply reporting serological data. For the most part, factual information such as the frequency of a particular blood group antigen has been omitted and reference is made to standard blood bank texts.

The educational design is flexible. As a result, it may be used as preparation for classroom instruction, in a classroom or by individuals who are studying independently.

We would like to express our appreciation to RMI Corporation of Cambridge, Massachusetts which was responsible for overall educational design and editing; preparation of illustrations, objectives and review questions; plus layout and paste-up.

Publication of this text would not have been possible without the assistance of Betty Hambleton. Her skill in operating word processing equipment was invaluable and she also suggested many changes to clarify meaning.

Finally, we thank Cora Sherry, our proofreader *par excellence*, who burned the midnight oil to meet our deadlines.

The following are trademarks of Ortho Diagnostic Systems Inc.:

AFFIRMAGEN Reagent Red Blood Cells

ANTIGRAM Antigen Profile

Blood Grouping Serum Anti-D (Anti-Rh_O) MAGNASERA for Slide and Rapid Tube Tests

Blood Grouping Serum Anti-D (Anti-Rh_O) NOVASERA for Saline Tube and Slide Tests

EluAid System for Antibody Elution

FETALDEX Quantitative Test for Fetal Red Blood Cells in the Maternal Blood Circulation

FETALSCREEN — A Qualitative Screening Test for D (Rh_O) Positive Fetal Red Blood Cells in the Maternal Circulation

MICRhoGAM Rh_O (D) Immune Globulin (Human) Micro-Dose

ORTHO A_2 Cells Reagent Red Blood Cells

ORTHO Anti-Human Serum (Rabbit)

ORTHO Anti-Human Serum (Rabbit) (Green)

ORTHO Blood Grouping Serum Anti-D (Anti-Rh_O) for Saline Tube Test

ORTHO Blood Grouping Serum Anti-D (Anti-Rh_O) for Slide and Modified Tube Tests

ORTHO Bovine Albumin Solution

ORTHO Bovine Albumin Solution — Polymerized Bovine Albumin

ORTHO Coombs Control Reagent Red Blood Cells

ORTHO Cord Cell Reagent Red Blood Cells

ORTHO Lewis Blood Group Substance

ORTHO Low Ionic Strength Solution (LISS)

ORTHO P_1 Blood Group Substance

ORTHO Pooled Screening Cells Reagent Red Blood Cells

ORTHO Reagent Confidence Sera

RESOLVE Panel A Reagent Red Blood Cells

RESOLVE Panel B Reagent Red Blood Cells

RhoGAM Rh_O (D) Immune Globulin (Human)

SELECTOGEN Reagent Red Blood Cells

SURGISCREEN Reagent Red Blood Cells

Table of Contents

To the Student

This text is organized into eight chapters. Preceding each chapter is a list of learning objectives which specify what you should know in order to perform competently in the blood bank.

Each chapter of the text is subdivided into a series of numbered *focus questions*. A *focus question* is designed to draw attention to the major topic discussed in that particular section. You should read the textual material in each focus question and refer to figures and tables as instructed.

Following each focus question is a programmed exercise, consisting of review questions covering the material in that section. Correct answers to the review questions are provided in the margin of the text. Prior to answering the questions, you should cover the answers with a mask. After completing all the questions in the section, you should then remove the mask and determine whether your responses were correct. You will learn the material most effectively if you attempt to answer the questions before checking the response column.

A convenient glossary of the terms shown in **boldface type**, an index keyed to the focus questions, and sources of additional information appear at the end of the text.

Introduction to Blood Groups

Red blood cell destruction (**hemolysis**) is a normal function of the body. Millions of red cells (**erythrocytes**) are produced each minute and, as their normal life span of approximately 120 days draws to an end, the spleen **sequesters** and destroys them and the body recycles those components which can be reused. In addition to the normal constant process of red cell destruction, there are abnormal circumstances in which the rate and amount of hemolysis are increased. Of most concern to blood bankers are conditions in which red cell destruction is caused by the action of **antibody**. This type of hemolysis — immune destruction — occurs in transfusion reactions, hemolytic disease of the newborn and autoimmune hemolytic disease.

Most hemolytic transfusion reactions result from the action of antibody in the patient's **serum** which is specific for a foreign **antigen** on infused red cells from a donor. Interaction of antibody with antigen on red cells results in accelerated destruction of the red cells by the body's protective mechanisms. Hemolytic disease of the newborn is also the result of immune destruction of red cells, but in this situation the baby's erythrocytes are destroyed by maternal antibodies.

With the exception of antibodies of the ABO system, the kinds of antibodies that cause transfusion reactions and hemolytic disease of the newborn are found almost exclusively in persons who have a prior history of transfusion and/or pregnancy. Red blood cells introduced intravenously as blood transfusions or when the placenta separates at the termination of pregnancy are perceived as foreign if they carry antigens different from those of the host. Antibodies to the antigens on the foreign red cells can be produced in the same way that the body's immune system responds to bacteria. With proper testing, however, much of the immunization which would result from indiscriminate transfusions can be avoided, and nearly all Rh immunization caused by fetal red blood cells entering the maternal circulation can be prevented by the proper administration of **Rh immune globulin**.

In addition, even when antibody production has occurred, immune destruction of transfused red cells can be avoided. Laboratory testing can reveal the transfusion candidate who has antibody, allowing the blood bank to provide red cells that do not contain the corresponding antigen. While laboratory testing can also reveal antibodies in pregnant women, unfortunately, destruction of the red cells of their babies cannot be prevented. This makes it even more critical that Rh immune globulin be administered in all circumstances when it can prevent the production of antibodies.

The third form of immune destruction is caused by the interaction of antibody with the person's own red cell antigens. This is called **auto-immune hemolytic anemia.** The mechanism of antibody production against one's own antigens ("self") is extremely complex and not fully understood, but the interaction of **autoantibody** with red cell antigen causes red cell destruction similar to that involved in transfusion reactions and hemolytic disease of the newborn.

The blood bank technologist has two objectives. First and foremost is the prevention of antigen-antibody interaction in the body; this is accomplished by identifying those patients who have an antibody and supplying blood which lacks the corresponding antigen. The second objective is to prevent antibody production. To the extent possible, exposure to foreign antigens on transfused cells must be avoided. When red cell transfusions are required, donor blood as nearly like the patient's blood as practical should be selected. When exposure to foreign antigen is inevitable, as is the case when Rh-incompatible fetal red blood cells enter the maternal circulation, the immune response to the **D (Rh_o)** antigen must be suppressed by administering Rh immune globulin to the mother. To fulfill both of these objectives, it is essential that blood bankers learn all they can about antigens, antibodies and their interactions, and then apply this knowledge to laboratory procedures and practices.

Blood Bank Tests

Many different blood group antigens are found on the surface of the red blood cells of every individual. These antigens, the products of inherited genes, exist in a unique combination in everyone except identical twins. **Blood grouping** is the process of testing red cells to determine which antigens are present and which are absent. It is standard practice to test for A, B and D (Rh_o) antigens and to perform tests for other antigens in selected cases.

When a person does not have a particular red cell antigen, his or her serum may contain an antibody to that antigen. Whether or not the antibody is present in the serum depends on whether the person's immune system has been previously challenged by, and responded to, that specific antigen or something very similar to it. The human body is constantly exposed to antigens in pollens, food, bacteria and viruses. Some of these "natural" antigens are apparently so similar to human **blood group antigens** that they stimulate almost every susceptible person to produce antibodies. Thus, certain antibodies are expected in the serum of anyone whose red cells lack the reciprocal antigen. This is especially true of the ABO system. The test for **expected antibodies** of the ABO blood group system is called **reverse grouping**.

Unexpected antibodies can be demonstrated in the sera of a small percentage of people. In all probability these people have been exposed to red cells which carry antigens unlike their own. This exposure to human red cells may have been via transfusion or fetal-maternal hemorrhage. Pretransfusion testing can minimize (but not eliminate) exposure to non-self blood group antigens, but it is impractical to test the recipient and donor for antigens other than those known to be of major significance. In most instances this testing is limited to A, B and D (Rh$_o$). Even though they may have a history of transfusion or pregnancy, most people do not have unexpected antibodies because of the pretransfusion matching that is done, the administration of Rh immune globulin, variability in the potency of different antigens, the number of foreign red cells received, and the variability of the immune response in each individual. **Antibody screening tests** are used to detect those people whose sera contain one or more unexpected antibodies.

Subsequent to its detection, an antibody must be identified so that its significance can be judged. Some antibodies are harmless in transfusion and pregnancy while others are extremely dangerous. Antibody identification tests define the specificity of the antibody, but whether an antibody will or will not cause destruction of red cells bearing the corresponding antigen depends on a number of conditions which will be discussed later in the book.

Donor units compatible with the patient in terms of ABO and Rh are selected. If an antibody has been detected in the recipient, further selection of donor units may be necessary, depending on the identification and significance of the antibody. Prior to transfusion, a **crossmatch** is performed as a final check for incompatibility. In this procedure the serum of the recipient is tested with the red blood cells of each prospective donor. The term "crossmatch" comes from the original method used to determine that a donor unit and a recipient were suitably matched. It included the **major** side of the match (patient serum and donor cells) and the **minor** side of the match (patient cells and donor serum). Hence the designation CROSSmatch. Because the minor part of the match is no longer considered necessary, the term "crossmatch" is less descriptive today, but is still widely used. Some workers began to use **compatibility test**, or "tests for evidence of serological incompatibility" instead of "major crossmatch." The concept of compatibility encompasses much more than the crossmatch alone. It should include all pretransfusion testing of both recipient and donor: ABO grouping, Rh typing, antibody screening and a test for hepatitis. Many workers believe the emphasis on compatibility testing should be from this broad point of view, but most also believe that the crossmatch is a necessary part of providing compatible blood.

Terminology

Unfortunately, blood group nomenclature is inconsistent from one system to another. There is some logic involved but the learner should also simply memorize certain rules. Two kinds of symbols are used for blood group antigens: a single letter in upper or lower case, or a two-letter combination with a superscript. Examples are: A, D, c, Fy^a and Le^b. Single letters were used in the early days of immunohematology but the terminology had to be changed as more antigens were discovered and their genetic control was elucidated. In most systems superscripts indicate an allelic relationship. For example, Fy^b is the product of a gene allelic to that producing Fy^a.

When antigens are tested for and found to be present, the antigen symbol is followed directly by a plus sign (such as D+) and, when absent, by a minus sign (such as K−). When results of tests for antigens denoted by symbols with superscripts are written, the superscript and the + or − are put within parentheses as in the following examples: Fy(a+), Jk(a−b+).

The prefix "anti" designates an antibody to the antigen which follows the prefix, e.g., anti-D, anti-Fy^a. This designation on the label of a vial of reagent serum indicates the specificity of the antibody in the reagent. A single antibody identified in the serum of a patient or donor is described in the same way, but a mixture of antibodies of different specificities is written with only one prefix, e.g., anti-Fy^a plus K. The recording method appropriate for each test will become clearer as each blood group is discussed.

Factors Which May Affect Test Results

As will be evident throughout this book, tests for blood group antigens and antibodies may be affected by physiological conditions existing in the patient or donor, and by conditions of the test system.

The nature of the sample being tested is one factor that should be considered. Red cell antigens are best preserved in blood to which an **anticoagulant** has been added. On the other hand some antibodies are better detected in serum than in plasma. This is because most anticoagulants bind calcium and magnesium ions which are required for the activation of complement by certain antigen-antibody interactions. Antibodies which are more readily detected because they bind complement may be missed if plasma is used. The freshness of the serum also influences antibody detection in certain cases since the age of serum relates to loss of complement activity.

The type of reagent used plays a major role in the kind of test results obtained. When considering the testing of red cells, it is important that the **blood grouping serum** selected be appropriate for the kind of specimens to be tested. For example, some patients have problems which preclude the use of certain **antisera** (antisera for slide and rapid tube procedures) because of constituents required in their manufacture. Commercially available **reagent red cells** can be obtained from individual donors or as pools of cells from more than one donor; each type of product serves a different purpose. In addition, the results of antibody detection and identification procedures are influenced by the additives used, as well as by the **anti-human serum** chosen. These technical variables will be discussed in more detail throughout the book.

The major factor affecting blood bank test results is technique. False positive or false negative results may be obtained if insufficient attention is given to the following: proper collection and handling of specimens; serum/cell ratios; red cell concentrations; suspending media; incubation times; speed and time of centrifugation; and the manipulation of the tubes and their contents while examining for **agglutination**. Controls designed to detect failures of the test system and/or the test operator are essential. An observant worker who understands what to expect from controls may be rewarded by finding an exceptional and especially interesting blood. New antigens and antibodies are discovered because someone notices unexpected test results. If controls show that the test system and the reagents are functioning properly, the unexpected result must indicate an abnormality in the blood sample being tested. Rare genes, cell membrane changes associated with disease or medication, and breakdown of **self-recognition** can all be reflected in blood bank tests.

The first chapter of this text describes inherited and acquired antigens, the immune response, and antigen-antibody interactions *in vitro*.

Chapter One:

Antigens and Antibodies and Their *In Vitro* Interaction

Objectives for Chapter One

Upon completion of this chapter you should be able to:

1.1 • **Define:**
- phospholipid
- amphipathic
- bilipid layer
- oligosaccharides
- glycoproteins
- glycolipids
- neutralizing substances

• **Describe the structure of the red blood cell membrane**

1.2 • **Explain the effect of each of the following on the immune response:**
- chemical structure of the antigen
- degree of foreignness of the antigen
- number of red cells introduced
- route of introduction of the antigen

1.3 • **Describe and graph the primary immune response**

• **Describe and graph the secondary immune response**

• **Define:**
- lectins
- hybridoma
- monoclonal antibodies

1.4 • **Explain the relationships among the following cells in the immune response:**
- macrophages
- B cells
- T cells
- plasma cells

1.5 • **Describe the molecular structures of IgG and IgM antibodies**

• **Define antibody specificity**

• **Discuss the effect of each of the following on antigen-antibody interactions:**
- temperature
- time and ionic concentration
- antigen density

1.6 • **Define the following:**
- sensitization
- incomplete antibodies
- agglutination
- lysis
- complement
- anti-human serum
- direct antiglobulin test
- indirect antiglobulin test
- zeta potential
- water of hydration

• **Describe the stages of blood group antigen-antibody interactions *in vitro***

1.1

What are blood group antigens?

Red Cell Antigens

The surface of the red blood cell consists of a **bilipid membrane** in which large protein molecules are embedded. The morphology of red blood cells is shown in Figure 1.1A. The shape of the cell, along with its deformability, is maintained by skeletal proteins lying on the internal side of the bilipid layer. Hemoglobin fills the space surrounded by this complex membrane. The biconcave-disc shape of the red blood cell maximizes the cell surface area.

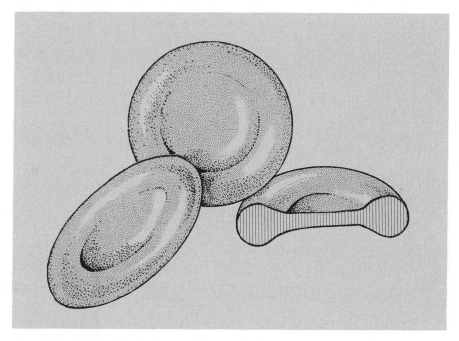

Figure 1.1A The morphology of red blood cells. Note the biconcave shape shown particularly in the cross-section of a cell at the bottom right.

The bilipid membrane is composed of a class of molecules called **phospholipids**, shown in Figure 1.1B. Phospholipids are **amphipathic**; that is, they have properties which are both **hydrophilic** and **hydrophobic**, as shown in Figure 1.1C. The polar heads of the molecules are hydrophilic and the hydrocarbon tails are hydrophobic. It is natural for phospholipids to form sheets or bilayers with the hydrophobic tails of each molecule sequestered within the bilipid layer. The hydrophilic heads are on the two surfaces of the bilipid layer — one surface exposed to the surrounding plasma while the other is exposed to hemoglobin. The membrane is asymmetric in that certain phospholipids dominate the outer layer (phosphatidylcholine and sphingomyelin) and others are predominantly on the inner layer (phosphatidylserine and phosphatidylethanolamine). The membrane is described as fluid because the lipid molecules actively migrate within the membrane parallel to the surfaces. They very rarely "flip-flop" from the outside to the inside or vice versa. This fluidity can be illustrated by showing that when two cells are fused their membranes completely integrate within about one hour.

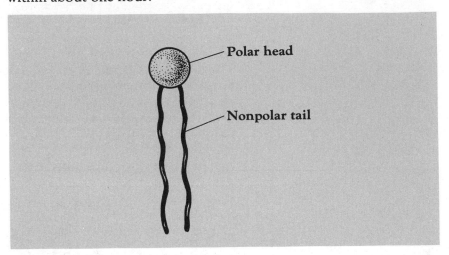

Figure 1.1B Illustration of a phospholipid which consists of a polar head and a nonpolar tail (two fatty acid side chains).

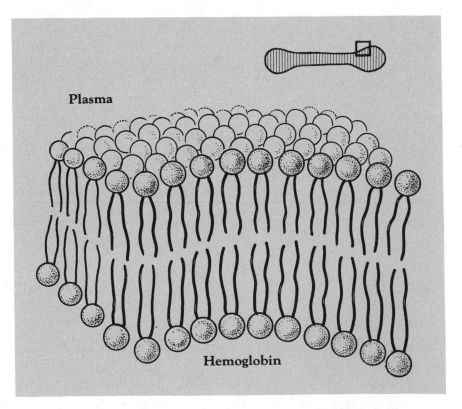

Figure 1.1C Illustration of the lipid bilayer of a red blood cell membrane. The large illustration is a magnification of a portion of the red blood cell membrane as indicated by the cutout (square) in the top right cross-sectional view of a red blood cell.

Most of the protein molecules in the bilipid membrane have **oligosac-charides** (groups of sugar molecules) attached in very precise positions. Some of these are known to be blood group antigens. Others serve as sites for metabolic functions of the red cell but have no recognized blood group specificity.

The most important blood group antigens are A, B and D (Rh$_0$). A and B antigens are well defined chemically. The antigenic determinants are the terminal sugars of oligosaccharide chains attached either directly to the cell membrane or attached to protein chains which protrude from the bilipid layer. When the oligosaccharide chains are attached to the cell membrane, the structure is called a **glycolipid** molecule, and when oligosaccharides are attached to a protein structure, the molecule is called a **glycoprotein**. The structure of the red blood cell membrane, including membrane proteins and oligosaccharides, is shown in Figure 1.1D. The Rh antigens are much less well defined but they are primarily protein and appear to be embedded in the bilipid membrane with portions of the molecule exposed on the outer surface of the cell. They are probably associated with one of the protein chains in the membrane which has already been partially characterized.

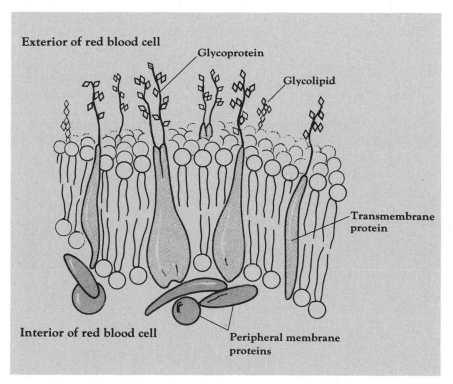

Figure 1.1D Illustration of the complex structure of a red blood cell membrane, including the proteins associated with the membrane. Transmembrane proteins span the width of the lipid bilayer from the exterior to the interior surface of the membrane. The sugar molecules (oligosaccharides) of these surface glycoproteins are indicated by the small diamond shapes. Also shown are glycolipids, that is, sugars attached directly to the bilipid layer. The glycolipids and some of the glycoproteins serve as blood group antigens. Peripheral membrane proteins on the interior surface of the membrane form a matrix which maintains the biconcave shape of the red blood cell.

The structure of all erythrocyte antigens is under strict genetic control. If a particular gene is inherited, the corresponding antigen is assembled and inserted into the membrane. Often a group of genes works in concert to produce a particular red blood cell antigen. The process of antigen production occurs during red blood cell maturation in the bone marrow prior to the loss of the red cell nucleus.

Non-Red-Cell Antigens

Some human body fluids contain soluble glycoproteins which have antigenic determinants identical with red cell antigens. When antigens are in solution the term **substance** is applied; thus, there are A and B antigens on red cells, and A and B substances in saliva and other body fluids. In addition to A and B substances, Lewis substances are also glycoproteins found in saliva and plasma. Lewis antigens are found on red cells also, but only because they have been taken up from the plasma.

Oligosaccharide chains like those associated with the surface of human red cells are also found in other forms of animal and plant life. For example, A, B and P antigens can be isolated from certain animal tissues, parasitic worms, pollens, bacteria and hydatid cyst fluid of sheep. Tissue-bound A, B and P antigens can be extracted and put into solution. These solubilized antigens, as well as the substances in body fluids from human or other sources, can be used to stimulate animals to produce antibodies for use as reagents. Blood group substances can also be made into reagents which neutralize the corresponding antibodies in human sera. Le^a, Le^b and P substances are available commercially. **Neutralizing substances** are very useful to the laboratory in identifying blood group antibodies.

1.1 QUESTIONS

The surface of a red blood cell consists of a:

☐ protein membrane.

☐ bilipid membrane.

☐ oligosaccharide membrane.

The normal shape of a red blood cell is:

☐ spherical.

☐ biconcave.

The red blood cell membrane is composed of a class of amphipathic molecules called _____ .

Amphipathic molecules are:

☐ hydrophilic.

☐ hydrophobic.

☐ both hydrophilic and hydrophobic.

The normal bilipid membrane is said to be fluid because the lipid molecules continually:

☐ "flip-flop" from the inside surface to the outside and vice versa.

☐ migrate within the plane of the membrane.

Oligosaccharides are groups of:

☐ protein molecules.

☐ lipid molecules.

☐ sugar molecules.

When oligosaccharide chains are attached to lipids, the complex molecules are called _____ .

When oligosaccharide chains are attached to proteins, the complex molecules are called _____ .

---

bilipid membrane.

biconcave.

phospholipids

both hydrophilic and hydrophobic.

migrate within the plane of the membrane.

sugar molecules.

glycolipids

glycoproteins

antigens

genetic control.

bone marrow.

A

B

D (Rh$_o$)

substances.

are

The terminal sugars of oligosaccharide chains on the surface of red blood cells often serve as blood group _____ .

The production of red blood cell antigens is under:

☐ genetic control.

☐ environmental control.

Antigen synthesis and insertion into the red blood cell membrane occur during red cell maturation usually in the:

☐ spleen.

☐ bone marrow.

☐ circulation.

List the three most important red cell antigens:

1 _____

2 _____

3 _____

Soluble glycoproteins which are identical to red cell antigenic determinants are called:

☐ substances.

☐ fragments.

☐ lectins.

Oligosaccharide chains resembling some red blood cell antigens

☐ are

☐ are not

found in other animal and plant life.

oligosaccharides found in human secretions and in other forms of animal and plant life which resemble red blood cell antigens. When substances combine with their corresponding antibodies, the antibodies are neutralized.

antibodies.

What are neutralizing substances?

_____

_____

_____

_____

_____

_____

Neutralizing substances are used in the laboratory to identify blood group:

☐ antibodies.

☐ antigens.

1.2

What factors affect immunogenicity?

Immunogenicity is a term used to describe the ability of an antigen to stimulate the production of its corresponding antibody in a person or animal that lacks the antigen.* Blood group antigens vary considerably in their immunogenicity. Therefore decisions concerning the extent of testing required prior to administering blood transfusions are based on an evaluation of these differences, as well as other considerations.

A comparative example will help to explain immunogenicity. The D antigen is a very effective immunogen. D negative persons transfused with D positive blood are very likely to produce anti-D. Therefore, testing must be done to prevent exposure to the D antigen whenever possible. In contrast, Fy^a is a poor immunogen. To provide Fy(a–) donors for all Fy(a–) recipients to prevent the production of anti-Fy^a would be a waste of time and resources.

Other factors that play a role in determining the extent of the immune response are listed below.

- **The chemical structure of the antigen**. Antigens which are primarily oligosaccharides tend to stimulate the production of a class of antibodies known as immunoglobulin M (**IgM**), while antigens which are primarily protein generally cause the production of **IgG**. Perhaps the position of the antigen on the red cell surface — whether it is more exposed or somewhat buried — also influences the degree of response to the antigen.

- **The degree of foreignness**. Even though a person lacks a particular antigen, his or her body may have proteins or carbohydrates that are similar to the antigen and these may prevent immunologic recognition. For example, porcine insulin is so similar to human insulin that most diabetics can be injected with it and not mount an immune response.

- **The number of red cells introduced and the amount of antigen they carry**. Even a very small number of red cells can cause immunization, but the risk increases as the quantity increases. In fact the significance may be more pronounced on the opposite end of the scale — a very large infusion of antigen may paralyze the immune response.

---

*Immunogen and antigen are synonymous. However, for the purpose of emphasis in this book, we will use the terms **immunogen** and **immunogenicity** when describing the ability of an antigen to stimulate the production of antibody *in vivo*.

- **The route of introduction**. Especially in animal experiments, the immune response varies depending on the quantity of antigen and whether the antigen is given intramuscularly, subcutaneously, etc. In humans this variation in effectiveness is reflected in the response to a large quantity of antigen introduced in a blood transfusion as compared to smaller quantities of fetal red blood cells which may enter the maternal circulation at intervals during pregnancy and at delivery.

Properties of the immunogen and the circumstances of the stimulus are not the only factors that influence the frequency with which a given antibody is observed. The frequency of the antigen in the population is especially significant. If only one person in thousands lacks a particular antigen and therefore is the only person who can produce the antibody, that antigen cannot be considered significant to the general population even though it may be an effective immunogen. A number of antigens that are nearly universal in the population (for example, k and Kp^b) are potent immunogens to the very rare person who lacks the antigen.

1.2 QUESTIONS

The ability of an antigen to stimulate the production of its corresponding antibody is called its _____ .

Match the following:

1 ____ D antigen	A	weak immunogen
2 ____ Fy^a antigen	B	strong immunogen

Match the following with respect to the effect of chemical structure in the immune response:

1 ____ antigens which are primarily oligo-saccharides	A	usually elicit an IgG response
2 ____ antigens which are primarily protein	B	usually elicit an IgM response

The greater the degree of foreignness of an antigen, the

☐ greater

☐ poorer

the immune response.

An immune response to a foreign red cell antigen usually requires the infusion of:

☐ only a small number of red cells.

☐ a rather large number of red cells.

Which route of introduction usually involves the larger number of red blood cells?

☐ blood transfusion

☐ transfer of red cells from the fetal to the maternal circulation during pregnancy and at delivery

Different blood group antigens vary significantly in their frequency in a given population.

Which of the following is correct?

☐ All blood group antigens are seen with approximately equal frequency in a given population.

☐ Different blood group antigens vary significantly in their frequency in a given population.

1.3

What are antibodies?

Antibodies can be recognized only by their interaction with antigens and vice versa. In the case of blood groups, this interaction is usually made visible by the agglutination of red cells. The characteristics of these interactions will be discussed in detail later in this chapter but the reader must first have an understanding of antibodies — what they are and how they originate.

Blood group antibodies are plasma proteins (specifically gamma globulin molecules) produced by the body as a defense mechanism in response to exposure to a foreign immunogen. The first time a person is exposed to a red cell antigen, the process by which the antigen is recognized as foreign or "non-self" is complex and therefore the response is slow. It may take two to six months before antibody is detectable. Antibody production in response to the first exposure to a foreign immunogen is called a **primary response**. A person may be "immunized" even though no antibody is detectable by common laboratory procedures. The graph in Figure 1.3A shows the approximate time course and relative antibody concentration of a primary response.

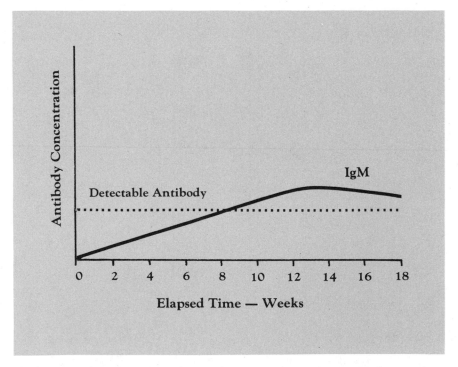

Figure 1.3A Graph of the time course of a primary immune response following the first challenge with an antigen. (Note: Time scale is in weeks, as compared to days in Figure 1.3B.)

If the person has mounted a primary response (whether antibody is demonstrable or not), a second exposure to the same immunogen will result in rapid production of large amounts of antibody. The antibody may be detectable in a few hours, a few days, or at most a few weeks. This **secondary response** is sometimes called an **anamnestic** (memory) response. Figure 1.3B is a graph of a secondary immune response.

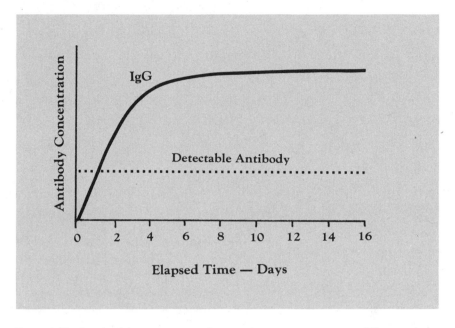

Figure 1.3B Graph of the time course of a secondary immune response following the second or subsequent challenges with the same antigen. (Note: Time scale is in days, as compared to weeks in Figure 1.3A.)

In addition to the time it takes to respond and the quantity of antibody produced, primary and secondary responses differ in the class of gamma globulin produced. In the primary response the antibody is usually IgM and in the secondary response the antibody is usually IgG. Simplified structures of IgG and IgM antibodies are shown in Figure 1.3C. The structures of these two antibodies are described in detail in Focus Question 1.5.

The presence of blood group antibodies is not always the result of exposure to red cell antigens. As mentioned previously, some chemical structures which are parts of plants and bacteria are similar to red cell antigens. Antibody produced in response to these non-erythrocyte immunogens is often referred to as **naturally-occurring antibody**. This is a misnomer but it is so well established in blood bank vocabulary that it is difficult to change. Antibodies never occur "naturally," i.e., spontaneously. They are always produced as an immune response to antigen; however, the source of the antigen may be the "natural" environment. In general, antibodies produced in response to non-erythrocyte immunogens resemble those of a primary response; i.e., the response is slow and the antibody is IgM. This holds true even though the exposure is continuous or repeated.

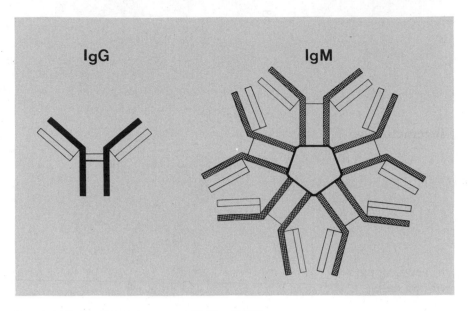

Figure 1.3C Simplified structures of IgG and IgM.

Antibodies from Animals and Plants

Human red blood cell antigens are foreign to other animals. Antibodies produced by animals when they are injected with human red blood cells or substances can be used in the manufacture of blood bank reagents. Rabbits and goats are chosen most often because they respond well to human immunogens, they are easy to handle, and they yield large volumes of serum.

There are also antibody-like materials in nature called **lectins** that react specifically with blood group antigens. Lectins are most commonly harvested from seeds but can also come from snails, horseshoe crabs, etc. Lectins are limited as reagents because only a few useful specificities have been found. However, lectins are especially valuable in the investigation of unusual blood types because of their very precise specificity.

A recent feat of modern science has been the development of a technique by which large quantities of antibodies can be made. This is accomplished by selecting specific antibody-producing spleen cells from an immunized mouse and fusing them with mouse **myeloma** cells. These fused cells, called **hybridomas**, are immortal antibody-producing cells which can be grown in culture media where they produce moderate quantities of antibody. Even more antibody can be harvested, however, by injecting the hybridoma cells into a mouse which develops peritoneal tumors that secrete antibody into the **ascites**. Very large quantities of antibody can be harvested from the ascites. Because the antibodies are made by a **clone** of cells derived from a single original cell, they are called **monoclonal antibodies**. All antibodies produced by a clone of cells are identical to each other in specificity, immunoglobulin class, and all other properties inherent in the original antibody-producing cell. Monoclonal antibodies can be especially useful when very precise specificity is needed in a reagent.

1.3 QUESTIONS

Blood group antigens can only be recognized by:

☐ observing their shape under a microscope.

☐ interaction with antibody.

☐ electrophoretic patterns.

Blood group antibodies are usually detected by:

☐ studying the immunogen used.

☐ observing agglutination of red cells.

Blood group antibodies are plasma:

☐ lipids.

☐ proteins.

☐ oligosaccharides.

Match the following:

1 _____ primary immune response   A   slow

2 _____ secondary immune response   B   rapid

A greater quantity of antibody is usually produced in the:

☐ primary immune response.

☐ secondary immune response.

Following a patient's first exposure to a foreign red cell antigen, approximately how much time is required before antibodies are detected in the patient's serum?

_____

In a secondary immune response, antibodies are detectable in the

serum within _____

_____ .

---

interaction with antibody.

observing agglutination of red cells.

proteins.

1 A

2 B

secondary immune response.

two to six months

a few hours, a few days, or at most a few weeks

<table>
<tr><td>

1 B

2 A

</td><td>

Match the following:

1 _____ primary immune   A IgG
        response

2 _____ secondary immune   B IgM
        response

</td></tr>
</table>

<table>
<tr><td valign="top" width="35%">

in response to exposure to plant or bacterial immunogens which resemble red cell antigens.

primary response.

foreign

red blood cells or substances

lectins

monoclonal

</td><td valign="top">

"Natural antibodies" are produced:

☐ spontaneously without exposure to any immunogen.

☐ in response to exposure to plant or bacterial immunogens which resemble red cell antigens.

Antibodies produced in response to non-erythrocyte immunogens are usually similar to those of a:

☐ primary response.

☐ secondary response.

Human red cell antigens are

☐ foreign

☐ not foreign

to most other animals.

Antibodies to human red cell antigens can be produced by injecting animals with human _____ .

Antibody-like materials found in nature which have a high degree of specificity for some human red cell antigens are called

_____ .

When a specific antibody-producing cell is fused with a myeloma cell, the result is a hybridoma which continues to divide and to produce

large quantities of _____ antibodies.

</td></tr>
</table>

1.4

What is the mechanism of the immune response?

The **immune response** is a complex interaction of antigen with **macrophages** and **lymphocytes**. The macrophage is stimulated by interaction with antigen and products of this interaction stimulate the lymphocytes. The lymphocytes involved can be divided according to their functional roles into **B cells** and **T cells**.

Macrophages are **phagocytic** cells which are either mobile or fixed in the loose connective tissue of the spleen, lymph nodes and liver. They have many roles in the body's immune defense mechanism, but the role of primary concern is that of capturing and processing antigens so that they can be presented to the B cells. (Macrophages also influence other parts of the immune system which are responsible for **allergic** and **inflammatory responses**. It is becoming evident that the macrophage plays a far greater role in the immune system than was previously believed.)

When a macrophage encounters foreign antigens such as bacteria or transfused red cells, the cell performs one of two functions: (1) it attracts the antigen which then adheres to the surface, allowing the macrophage to serve as a stage for the interaction of the antigen and the appropriate B cell, or (2) the macrophage ingests the cell (or part of it), processes the antigen, extrudes it and holds the antigen on the surface until the antigen is recognized by a B cell.

B cells are the factories which produce antibody. The designation "B" comes from the word **bursa**, an organ in chickens which processes precursor lymphocytes into cells which have the potential to produce antibodies. There is no organ in man known to serve this role, but the term "B cell" is used to describe cells which have the same potential to produce antibodies.

Unlikely as it seems, there are a few B cells (a single clone of cells) programmed by **genetic code** to produce antibody against every conceivable antigen. The recognition of antigen by the "committed" B cell is accomplished by receptor sites on the surface of the B cell. These receptors are (or closely resemble) antibody molecules. When one of the few committed B cells encounters the antigen (captured by a macrophage), various signals are received and the antibody-producing cycle is put into motion. The B cell enlarges, loses the surface receptors and develops a complex internal structure which starts to produce antibody of the same specificity as the surface receptor. In this stage the cells are called **plasma cells**. Each of the plasma cells produces vast quantities of antibody of the precise specificity and immunoglobulin class genetically programmed into the cell. The cells also proliferate so that millions of antibody molecules are produced every minute.

Besides the physical presentation of the antigen to the B cell, the antigen-bearing macrophage also stimulates T cells to proliferate. The designation "T" comes from the word **thymus**, the organ which processes precursor lymphocytes (called **thymocytes**) into functioning T cells. The roles played by T cells are even more diverse than those associated with either macrophages or B cells. In relation to their interaction with B cells, T cells fall into two broad categories (helper and suppressor) which regulate the type and intensity of the immune response. When a specific helper T cell physically interacts with an antigen-bearing macrophage, the T cell proliferates and the cells produce substances (not to be confused with blood group substances) which in turn stimulate the proliferation of antibody-producing B cells. In other words, following stimulation by antigen, macrophages, B cells and T cells have interlocking functions. The processing of antigens by macrophages and their subsequent interaction with B cells and T cells is shown in Figure 1.4A.

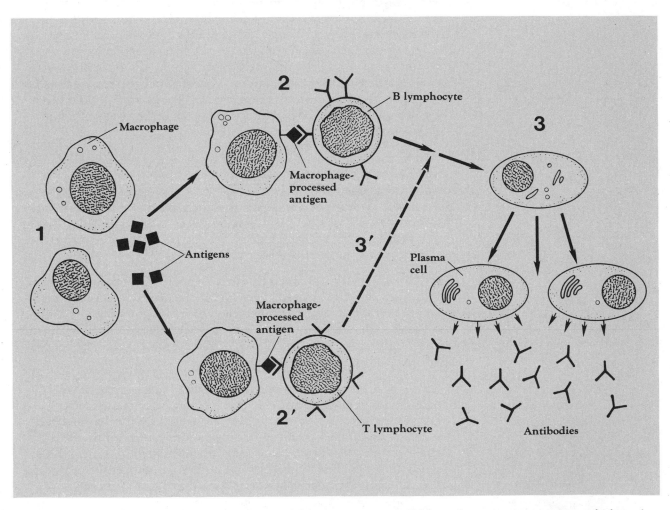

Figure 1.4A The immune response. (1) Macrophages encounter antigens, which are then processed by the macrophages and "presented" to B cells (2) and T cells (2′). As a result of B cell interaction with antigen-bearing macrophages, B cells differentiate into plasma cells (3), which produce antibodies. T cells proliferate as a result of interaction with antigen-bearing macrophages. T cells can either help or suppress (3′) B cell differentiation into plasma cells.

It is currently believed that if an antigen-bearing macrophage encounters a committed B cell but not the corresponding T cell, the B cell responds by making IgM antibody. Under these circumstances the B cell proliferates slowly, but if one or more of the IgM-producing B cells interacts with the appropriate helper T cell, a portion of the genetic code of the B cell is turned off and another portion is turned on. The new message instructs the cell to make IgG antibody of the same specificity. This "switching" of genetic message may help to explain the differences between the primary response to antigen, which is slow and usually IgM, and the secondary response of the same specificity, which is rapid and usually IgG.

1.4 QUESTIONS

What are the three types of cells involved in the immune response?

macrophages

1 _____

B lymphocytes (B cells)

2 _____

T lymphocytes (T cells)

3 _____

Which of the above types of cells can develop into antibody-secreting cells?

B cells

_____

Such antibody-producing cells are called:

☐ macrophages.

plasma cells.

☐ plasma cells.

☐ both

The antigen receptors present on the surface of B cells are (or closely

antibody molecules

resemble) _____ .

Each plasma cell produces antibodies with:

☐ one precise specificity.

one precise specificity.

☐ multiple specificities.

Macrophages are important in capturing and

☐ destroying

processing

☐ processing

antigens.

In the immune response, antigen-bearing macrophages can interact with:

☐ B cells.

☐ T cells.

☐ both

both

Precursor thymocytes mature into functional T cells in which organ?

☐ spleen

☐ thymus gland

☐ bone marrow

thymus gland

The two broad categories of T cells are:

☐ helper and suppressor T cells.

☐ antibody-producing and antibody-processing T cells.

helper and suppressor T cells.

It is currently hypothesized that when a committed B cell interacts with an appropriate antigen-bearing macrophage but *not* with a corresponding T cell, the B cell develops into a plasma cell producing

_____ antibodies.

IgM

If the above B cell interacts with an appropriate helper T cell, it would then develop into plasma cells producing

☐ IgG

☐ IgM

antibodies.

IgG

1.5

What concepts must be considered in relation to *in vitro* antigen-antibody interactions?

As stated in the Introduction, the primary objective of the transfusion service is to prevent the administration of red blood cells with a particular antigen to a person whose serum contains an antagonistic antibody. Since antibodies of the ABO system are expected to be present, selection of ABO-compatible donors is essential for all blood transfusions. Fortunately, most people have not been further immunized by exposure to foreign red blood cells. However, to recognize those who *have* been immunized, *in vitro* testing is done. Serum is tested with red cells of known antigen makeup (reagent red cells) and there will be some observable reaction if the serum contains antibody specific for one or more of the antigens on the cells. Antibodies react in a variety of ways and, since there is no way of knowing which antibody may be present, conditions to satisfy the needs of any significant antibody must be provided. Certain concepts that must be considered include the molecular structure of antibodies, antibody specificity, test milieu, and antigen density and accessibility.

The Structure of Antibodies

Plasma proteins can be separated into various components by different techniques. The proteins of major concern to blood bankers are **fibrinogen**, **albumin** and **globulins**. Fibrinogen is one of the major components of the coagulation system necessary for the clotting of blood. Albumin serves a number of functions. One of these is to combine with **bilirubin** to form an excretable complex. Maintaining water balance and controlling the viscosity of plasma, both of which are essential for normal blood pressure, are other functions of albumin. Globulins can be further divided into many subcomponents of which **beta** and **gamma globulins** are of particular interest. Since all gamma globulins are related to the immune response, gamma globulins are now more commonly designated **immunoglobulins**, often abbreviated to Ig. Immunoglobulins can also be divided into three categories: IgG, IgM and IgA. Most blood group antibodies fall into one of two categories — IgM or IgG — but occasionally some antibody is IgA. IgG can be subclassified according to structure and function into IgG1, IgG2, IgG3 and IgG4. Some properties of immunoglobulins are given in Table 1.5A.

Table 1.5A Properties of human immunoglobulins.

	IgG	IgA	IgM
H chain, class	γ	α	μ
Molecular weight	150,000	180,000-500,000	900,000
Electrophoretic mobility	γ	slow γ	between γ and β
Carbohydrate percentage	2.6	5-10	9.8
Serum concentration (mg/dL)	1000-1500	200-350	85-205
Secretion	No	Yes	No
Fixes complement	Occasionally	No	Yes
Crosses placenta	Yes	No	No

Molecular Structure

All proteins are made of amino acid molecules joined by **peptide bonds**. Amino acids joined in this manner are called **amino acid** residues and the chains formed are called **polypeptide chains**. Polypeptide chains may assume various configurations. They may be linear sequences of amino acid residues, they may be folded into globular formations, or they may combine with other polypeptide chains to form complex protein molecules. The final conformation is dependent on the sequence of amino acids in the primary chains. The sequence of amino acids in immunoglobulins (antibodies) is regulated by the genes of the antibody-producing B cell.

The IgG molecule is made up of 1200-1500 amino acid residues and has a molecular weight of about 150,000 daltons. As shown in Figure 1.5B, an IgG molecule is composed of four chains — two identical heavy chains (**H chains**) and two identical light chains (L chains) — joined together by covalent disulfide bonds and noncovalent bonds. The terminal portions of one H chain and one L chain function together when the antibody combines with its corresponding antigen. The ability to combine with antigen is dependent on only a few of the amino acid residues at the end of each chain. The antibody molecule can be reduced to smaller fragments, allowing closer study of its structure. The fragment or portion that retains the ability to combine with antigen consists of all the L chain and some of the H chain and is called the **Fab piece** (Fragment antigen binding). The remainder of the molecule, composed of pieces of both H chains, is called the **Fc piece** (Fragment crystallizable) because it can be crystallized. The sites for other functions of the molecule, such as complement fixation, placental transport and reaction with anti-human serum, reside on the Fc piece.

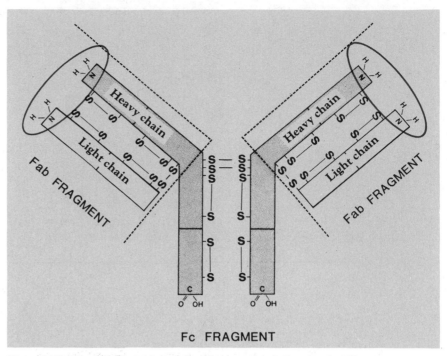

Figure 1.5B Detailed illustration of the structure of an IgG molecule. Areas shown within the ovals indicate the antigen-binding sites.

The **hinge region**, where the L chain attaches to the H chain, is so named because it is at this point that the molecule can bend or open and close under different conditions. When fully open, the distance from one antigen-binding site to the other is about 240 Å (24 nm). This explains why an antibody is unable to combine with more than one antigen on a given red cell. Although the red cell is about 7000 nm in diameter, few blood group antigens are so abundant under normal conditions to be within 24 nm of each other. A and B antigens are exceptions.

IgM molecules (about 900,000 daltons) are larger than IgG molecules and are composed of five subunits which resemble five IgG molecules (see Figure 1.3C). However, the H chains differ from those of IgG, and an IgM molecule is *not* simply five IgG molecules joined together. The maximum distance spanned by two antigen-binding sites of IgM is about 420 Å (42 nm). Other differences between IgG and IgM will be discussed later in the book.

Antibody Specificity

The concept of **specificity** is primary to an understanding of antigen-antibody interaction. When the body recognizes an antigen as foreign and produces an antibody against it, the antibody is specific for that antigen and will not interact with other antigens. As shown in Figure 1.5C, specificity is dependent on how well the antigen "fits" the antigen-binding site (Fab) of the antibody and on the number of electrostatic charges at the site of interaction which bind the antigen and antibody together. Being proteins and/or carbohydrates, blood group antigens carry characteristic patterns of positive and negative charges.

Antibodies are proteins which also carry positive and negative charges. The unlike charges of the antigen and antibody attract, and a bond is formed. The affinity of the antibody for its antigen is directly proportional to the conformational fit and to the number of unlike charge pairs within the structure of the antigen-antibody complex.

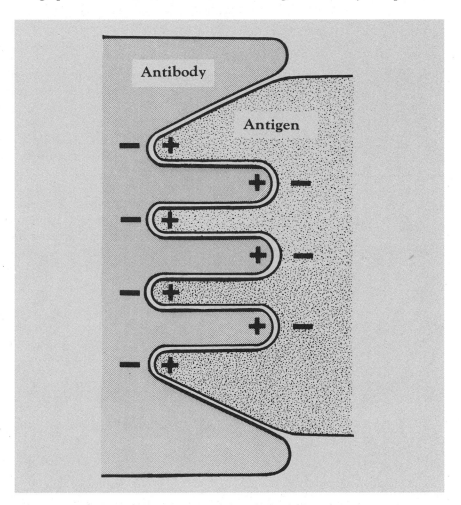

Figure 1.5C Schematic illustration of antibody specificity showing the complementary interaction of the charge groups of the antigen and antibody molecules.

Like all minute particles in suspension, red cells and antibodies are in constant motion even during *in vitro* testing. Whether or not the antibody encounters its antigen on the red cell is almost totally based on chance. When an antigen and antibody bind together, the bonds are not permanent but reach a state of dynamic equilibrium under given conditions. This is expressed by the following equation:

$$Ag + Ab \underset{k_2}{\overset{k_1}{\rightleftharpoons}} AgAb$$

At equilibrium, the rate of formation of antigen-antibody complexes (k_1) equals the rate of dissociation of antigen-antibody complexes (k_2); i.e., at equilibrium $k_1 = k_2$. The time it takes to reach equilibrium can be altered by increasing or decreasing temperature and by changing the ionic concentration of the reaction environment.

Test Milieu

Conditions of the test milieu that should be considered include temperature, time and ionic concentration, and antigen density.

Temperature

When tested in the laboratory, most significant antibodies react optimally at 37°C (body temperature) and are described as **warm antibodies**. Some antibodies exhibit stronger reactivity below body temperature and are referred to as **cold antibodies**. The thermal ranges of "warm" and "cold" antibodies are illustrated in Figure 1.5D. Antibodies which react only below 30°C are not clinically significant because they do not react at normal body temperature. The more strongly reactive a cold antibody, the wider the temperature range over which it reacts. Many people believe that testing at room temperature for antibodies other than those of the ABO system only creates confusion. Significant warm antibodies will not go undetected if room temperature tests are omitted because they will react in other phases of the test procedure. Cold antibodies that react at room temperature but not in the range of 30°C to 37°C should not be dignified by the use of resources needed to identify them.

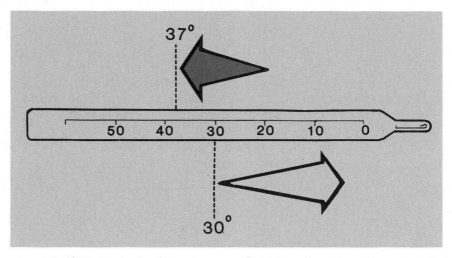

Figure 1.5D Illustration of the thermal ranges of warm antibodies reacting optimally at 37°C and cold antibodies reacting only at temperatures below 30°C.

Time and Ionic Concentration

At its optimum temperature, the rate at which an antibody attaches to its specific antigen depends largely on the ionic strength of the reaction milieu. This varies with the suspending medium used for the red cells and the additives or **potentiators** incorporated into the test system (either in reagents or added as part of the test procedure).

Traditionally, the integrity of red cells has been maintained by suspending them in isotonic salt solutions (saline, ACD, CPDA-1, etc.). Saline (NaCl) ionizes in solution producing Na^+ and Cl^- ions and these ions cluster around the red cell. When an antibody and antigen of complementary electrostatic charge interact, some of these Na^+ and Cl^- ions "get in the way" and must be pushed aside before a tight bond can be formed. Solutions in which the concentrations of Na$^+$ and Cl$^-$ are lower than normal saline are called **low ionic strength solutions**, abbreviated LISS. In such solutions, the interaction of the antigen and antibody proceeds more rapidly. The presence of **bovine albumin** influences mainly red cell agglutination (the second stage of antigen-antibody interaction). The effect of time and ionic concentration on antigen-antibody reactions is illustrated in Figure 1.5E.

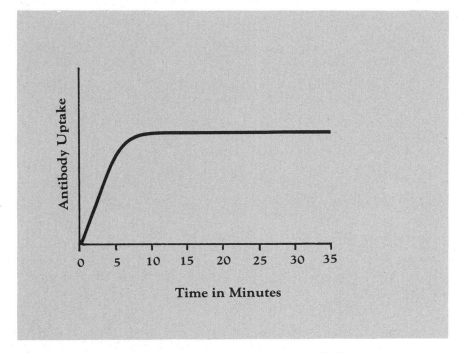

Figure 1.5E The effect of time on antibody uptake at a final ionic concentration of 0.09 M.

Antigen Density

How an antibody combines with its antigen and whether or not there is any visible effect on the red cell depend not only on the specificity of the particular antibody involved and the constituents of the test milieu but also on the density of the antigen on the cell.

The density of antigen and its availability to the antibody may play a greater role than was previously realized. Figure 1.5F is an illustration of antigen density. There is little question that the rapid and strong reactions observed in tests using anti-A and anti-B reagents reflect the density of the antigens (about one million per cell) as much as the properties of the antibody. Characteristically, IgM agglutinates red blood cells in saline, whereas IgG requires the addition of a potentiator such as bovine albumin. Most probably the agglutination of A and B cells observed when testing the serum of cord bloods (in which the anti-A and anti-B are IgG) is due to the large number of antigens on the cell. The M and N antigens are also very abundant on red cells (500,000 per cell) and this density of antigen contributes to the ability of IgG anti-M to cause agglutination in saline.

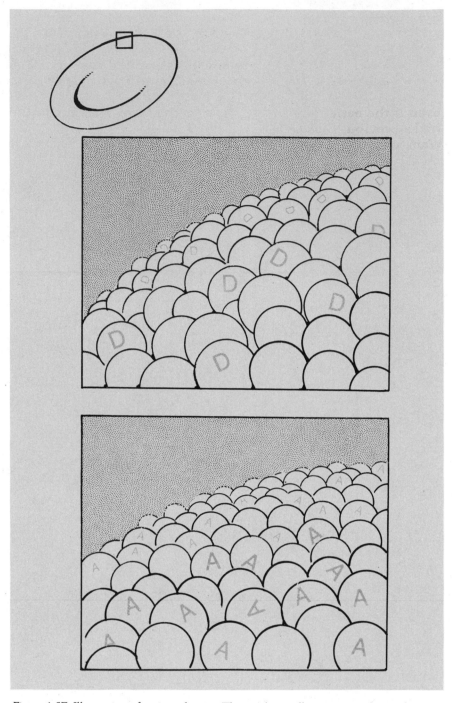

Figure 1.5F Illustration of antigen density. The two larger illustrations are magnifications of the cutout (square) at the top left. As shown, the A antigen has a much higher antigen density on the surface of the red blood cell than does the D antigen. There are about 20 times more A (or B) antigen sites than D antigen sites.

Antibodies of the ABO system are expected to be present in a patient:

☐ even if the patient has not had a previous blood transfusion.

☐ only if the patient has had a previous blood transfusion.

Match the following for the plasma proteins:

1 ___ fibrinogen	A	important in the maintenance of water balance and the viscosity of plasma
2 ___ albumin	B	includes blood group antibodies
3 ___ globulins	C	an important component of the coagulation system

Most blood group antibodies fall into which two immunoglobulin classes?

_____

Antibodies are primarily:

☐ proteins.

☐ lipids.

☐ carbohydrates.

An IgG antibody is composed of how many heavy chains and how many light chains?

____ heavy chains

____ light chains

Match the following:

| 1 ___ binds to antigens | A | Fab piece |
| 2 ___ site of complement fixation, placental transport, and reaction with anti-human serum | B | Fc piece |

---

even if the patient has not had a previous blood transfusion.

1 C

2 A

3 B

IgG and IgM

proteins.

two

two

1 A

2 B

hinge region	The region of the IgG antibody where the antibody can open or bend is called the _____.
five	The structure of an IgM molecule consists of ☐ three ☐ five ☐ ten subunits.
conformational fit and the number of unlike charge pairs	The specificity of an antibody for its corresponding antigen depends on _____ _____.
reversible event.	The binding of an antigen and antibody is a(n) ☐ reversible event. ☐ irreversible event.
can	The temperature and ionic concentration of the reaction medium ☐ can ☐ cannot alter the time it takes for an antigen-antibody reaction to reach equilibrium.
37	Warm antibodies react optimally at _____ degrees centigrade.
30	Cold antibodies usually react only below _____ degrees centigrade.
rapidly	Antigen-antibody reactions proceed more ☐ rapidly ☐ slowly in low ionic strength solutions than in normal saline.

high

Rapid and strong antigen-antibody reactions often reflect a

☐ high

☐ low

antigen density on red blood cells.

1.6

What are the stages of antigen-antibody interaction?

Red Cell Sensitization

Many blood group antibodies combine with their corresponding antigens on red cells *in vitro* and do not themselves cause any observable change. These antibodies are IgG molecules which attach only one Fab piece to an antigen site on the red cell. The other Fab piece remains free and, because of the distance between cells, cannot attach to the antigen of a different cell. As seen in Figure 1.6A, agglutination does not occur. Antibodies that do not agglutinate cells directly have been called **incomplete antibodies** or **sensitizing antibodies**, and red cells that have such antibodies on their surfaces are called **sensitized cells**. Making the antigen-antibody interaction observable requires either the antiglobulin technique or the use of solutions that change the test milieu.

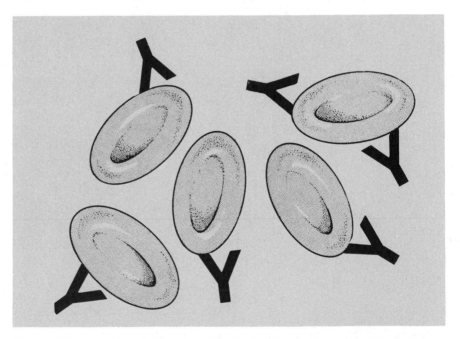

Figure 1.6A Illustration of red cell sensitization by IgG. As shown, sensitized cells have antibodies attached to their surfaces by only one binding site.

Another observable phenomenon which may result from red cell antigen-antibody interaction is **lysis** of the cell (hemolysis). This requires the cooperation of another defense mechanism of the body — the **complement system**. Complement components are normal body proteins, mainly beta globulins. **Complement fixation** is a series of enzymatic reactions, each one activated by the product of the reaction before it. The initial step of complement activation is triggered by antibody which has attached to antigen, but only some antibodies have the ability to activate the complement system. When certain blood group antibodies attach to a red cell, conformational changes occur in the antibody molecule. This change in shape allows the first component of complement to attach to the antibody. This attachment initiates a series of enzymatic reactions within the complement system in which some of the complement components (especially C3) attach directly to the cell membrane. The final components in the sequence of reactions (C5, C6, C7 and C8) combine to form lesions in the membrane and the cell is destroyed. This is illustrated in Figure 1.6B. The red color of free hemoglobin released during the immune destruction of red cells (in addition to or instead of agglutination) indicates an antigen-antibody interaction must have taken place. The observation of hemolysis during antibody detection procedures is as important as the observation of agglutination. Antibodies that fix complement are usually IgM, but occasionally they are IgG.

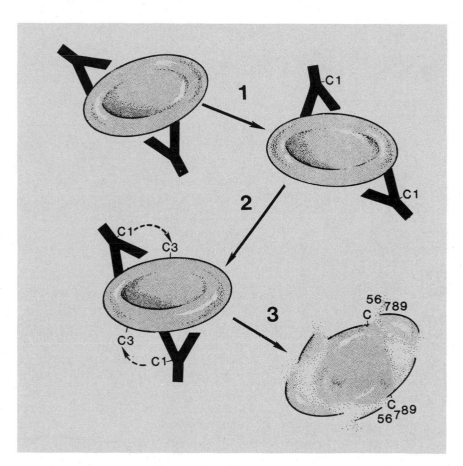

Figure 1.6B Illustration of complement-mediated red blood cell lysis. (1) Antibodies bound to red cells activate complement. In order to activate complement a pair of antibodies must be bound to the cell in close proximity to each other. (Only one is shown.) The first component, C1, binds to a receptor in the Fc region, which becomes accessible when the shape of the antibody is altered as a result of binding to antigen. (2) Through a series of enzymatic reactions (illustrated by the dotted line), C3 is bound to the surface of the red cells. (3) If complement activation proceeds to completion, C5, 6, 7, 8 and 9 penetrate the membrane and lysis results.

As seen in Table 1.6C, complement fixation does not always proceed through the entire sequence of steps to cause lysis of red cells. For reasons not entirely understood, the process often stops after the first few steps, leaving some complement components fixed to the cell but with no observable lysis. Depending on whether the antigen-antibody interaction occurs *in vivo* or *in vitro*, either C3b or C3d will be the final component on the cell surface. Very small quantities of antibody are needed to initiate complement fixation — often too small to cause agglutination — but the C3b or C3d fixed by the antibody can be detected in the antiglobulin test if suitable anti-human serum is used.

Table 1.6C Steps in the complement/anti-complement antiglobulin test.

1. Complement-fixing antibodies attach to red cell antigens.

2. The first component of complement (C1) is made up of three parts: C1q, C1r and C1s. C1q is bound to the Fc piece of each of a pair of IgG molecules. (If the antibody is IgM, only one molecule is required.)

3. The attachment of C1q converts C1s to an active enzyme $\overline{C1s}$. (The bar over the symbol denotes an *active* enzyme.)

4. $\overline{C1s}$ cleaves C4. C4b, a major fragment of C4, binds directly to the red cell surface. $\overline{C1s}$ also fragments C2.

5. Fixed C4b complexes with C2a, a fragment of C2, producing $\overline{C4b2a}$.

6. The $\overline{C4b2a}$ complex, called C3 convertase, cleaves C3 into C3a and C3b, and large amounts of C3b are bound directly to the red cell surface.

7. C3b is detectable by suitably prepared anti-human serum.

In vivo C3b is further acted upon to produce C3d. C3d is the complement component found on cells drawn from patients with conditions that activate complement *in vivo*. Anti-human serum specific for C3d is available.

Anti-Human Serum and the Antiglobulin Test

The immune response is a characteristic limited to vertebrates. As stated previously, the ability to produce antibodies to a foreign antigen is directly proportional to the degree of "foreignness." Whereas insulin molecules are very similar in structure whether they are from pigs, cows or humans, serum proteins such as albumin or globulins differ somewhat in different species. These differences are readily recognized by an animal injected with the albumin or globulins from another species, and antibodies are produced. Rabbits injected with human gamma globulin produce anti-human gamma globulin, and their serum can be made into anti-human globulin serum — one of the most useful reagents in blood banks and transfusion services.

Anti-human serum is made from the serum of rabbits immunized with purified human serum components, i.e., gamma globulin or beta globulin. Ideally, separate rabbit colonies are used in the preparation of anti-human serum. As shown in Figure 1.6D, one colony is injected with purified human IgG and these rabbits produce antibodies specific for gamma globulin (anti-IgG). Another colony of rabbits is injected with purified human beta globulin, as shown in Figure 1.6E, and these rabbits produce antibodies specifically against the beta globulins, i.e., complement components of human serum.

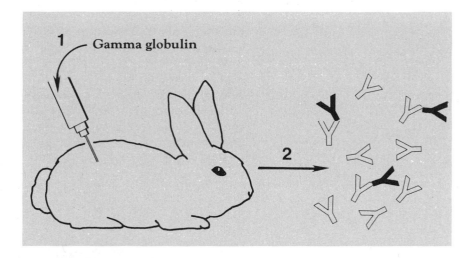

Figure 1.6D The production of anti-human serum. (1) Purified human gamma globulin is injected into a rabbit. (2) The rabbit's immune system recognizes the human IgG as foreign and produces anti-human IgG (shown in outline).

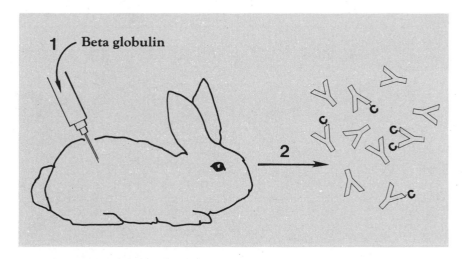

Figure 1.6E The production of anti-human serum specific for complement. (1) Purified human beta globulin is injected into the rabbit. (2) The rabbit's immune system recognizes the human beta globulin as foreign and produces antibodies which react specifically with complement, the only beta globulin likely to be on the cell surface.

After absorption to remove unwanted antibodies, the two kinds of rabbit antibodies are combined to produce polyspecific anti-human serum — a blend of anti-IgG and anti-complement which will react with red cells sensitized with antibody and/or complement. The preparation of monospecific anti-human serum requires processing of the rabbit sera from each individual colony rather than combining them to make polyspecific anti-human serum.

The principle of the antiglobulin test is simple. Unattached serum globulin is removed from around the sensitized red cells and anti-human serum is added. (If unattached globulins are not removed, they will combine with and neutralize the anti-human serum and a false negative test may result.) The rabbit anti-IgG molecules attach by their Fab pieces to the Fc pieces of the human sensitizing antibody, resulting in agglutination of the red cells. The agglutination of IgG-sensitized red blood cells by anti-human serum is shown in Figure 1.6F. In a similar manner, after complement-sensitized cells are freed of unattached globulins, rabbit anti-complement attaches to the complement components and, since complement components are attached to the red blood cells, agglutination results. The agglutination of complement-sensitized red blood cells by anti-human serum is shown in Figure 1.6G.

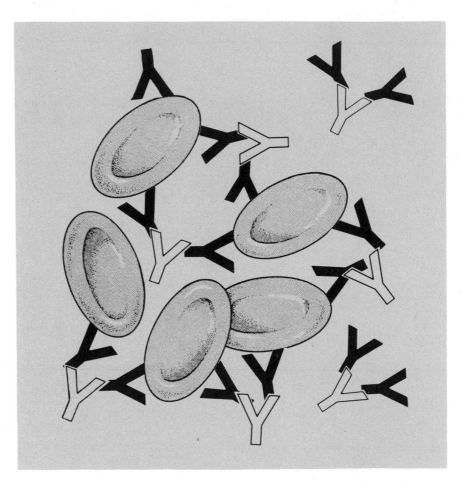

Figure 1.6F Illustration of IgG-sensitized red blood cells agglutinated by anti-human serum. The solid molecules are the blood group antibodies while the outlined molecules are the anti-human serum antibodies. If unattached globulins are not removed, they will combine with and neutralize the anti-human serum and a false negative test may result.

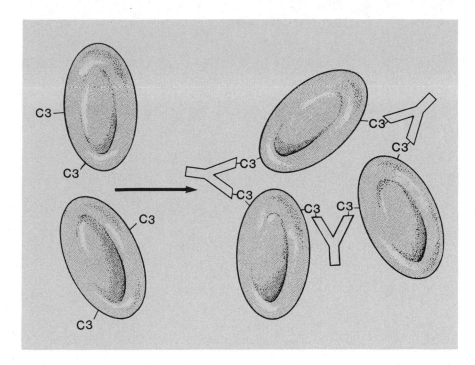

Figure 1.6G Illustration of the agglutination of complement-sensitized red cells by anti-human serum.

By convention any test which incorporates anti-human serum is called an **antiglobulin test**. It is essential to understand the difference between direct and indirect antiglobulin tests. Under normal circumstances antibody is never attached to red cells in the body. It is only in the conditions mentioned earlier — autoimmune hemolytic anemia, hemolytic disease of the newborn and transfusion reactions — that antibody is attached to red cells *in vivo*. Detection of *in vivo* sensitization requires only removal of unattached globulin and the addition of anti-human serum. The procedure just described is called the **direct antiglobulin test** or direct Coombs test (Dr. R.R. Coombs, a veterinarian, developed the test in 1945).

When a person has antibodies but there are no red cells present that carry the corresponding antigen, the antibodies circulate freely. These antibodies can be detected by testing serum *in vitro* with reagent red cells and observing agglutination of the cells following the addition of anti-human serum. Testing for antibodies in this indirect way is called the **indirect antiglobulin test**. This term can be applied to a variety of procedures such as antibody detection, antibody identification and the crossmatch. In addition, the indirect antiglobulin test can be used to identify an unknown antigen when antibody of known specificity is used (as in blood grouping with reagent antisera). The indirect antiglobulin test is illustrated in Figure 1.6H.

The indirect antiglobulin test will detect the vast majority of IgG blood group antibodies, being limited only by the amount of antibody fixed to the red cells. Under certain test conditions, however, IgG of some specificities (especially Rh) will cause red cells to agglutinate before the washing phase of the antiglobulin procedure.

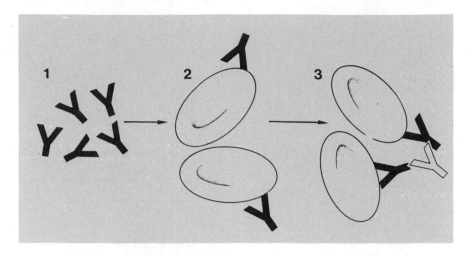

Figure 1.6H The indirect antiglobulin test. (1) Serum containing blood group antibodies. The blood group antibodies may be from transfusion candidates, obstetrical patients or donors, or they may be from reagent sera. (2) Red cells are added to the serum and are sensitized after a period of time. The red cells may be reagent red cells or may be from a patient or donor. (3) The sensitized red cells are agglutinated by the anti-human serum (shown in outline).

Intercellular Forces and Agglutination

We have discussed red cell sensitization by IgG antibody molecules and the subsequent detection of those antibodies by reacting the cells with anti-human serum and observing agglutination. Under other circumstances agglutination of red cells is a direct result of the attachment of antibody. This is universally true of IgM antibodies, but some IgG antibodies will also agglutinate red cells if certain conditions are provided.

Even though red cell agglutination was observed before 1900, we do not yet have a thorough understanding of the forces involved. There are two current theories, neither of which accounts for all observations. Parts of both theories may be correct or a new theory may replace all or most of our current explanations. Whatever the explanation may prove to be, we know that we can cause some incomplete or non-agglutinating antibodies to agglutinate red cells by either changing the reaction medium in which the cells are suspended or altering the cell membrane.

The zeta potential theory states that the natural tendency for cells to aggregate is offset by forces of repulsion which determine the minimum distance between cells. If this distance is too great, no agglutination can occur because small antibody molecules cannot bridge the cells. The average minimum distance between the cells can be decreased by reducing the forces of repulsion.

Red cells in solution are in constant random thermal motion. The minimum distance is maintained by the strong net negative surface charge of the cells. As the cells move about randomly, they can approach each other only to within a certain distance before the forces of repulsion (like charges repel) push the cells apart. The negative charge is derived mainly from the large number of sialic acid residues (N-acetylneuraminic acid) attached to protein chains embedded in the bilipid membrane of the red cell.

A cloud of ions surrounds each cell when red blood cells are suspended in saline. Positively charged ions (Na^+) are attracted to the negatively charged cell surface, and negatively charged ions (Cl^-) diffuse outward, forming an "atmosphere" around the cell. The surface at which this cloud of ions ceases to "travel with" the cell is known as the **surface of shear** or the **slipping plane**. This is the effective surface of the cell in relation to the approach of another cell. When the slipping plane of one cell approaches the slipping plane of another, the like negative charges of the cells repel and oppose any further motion toward each other.

The electric potential measured between the cell membrane and the slipping plane is known as **zeta potential**. Zeta potential is calculated by a formula which takes into account viscosity, the electrophoretic mobility of the cell and the dielectric constant of the suspending medium. By controlling these factors, the zeta potential can be altered and the minimum distance can be controlled. Agglutination of red cells by IgG is shown in Figure 1.6I. When cells are suspended in saline, IgM antibodies can bridge the cells by attaching to their specific antigens, but the minimum separation distance is too great for IgG antibodies to span. Agglutination of red cells by IgM is shown in Figure 1.6J.

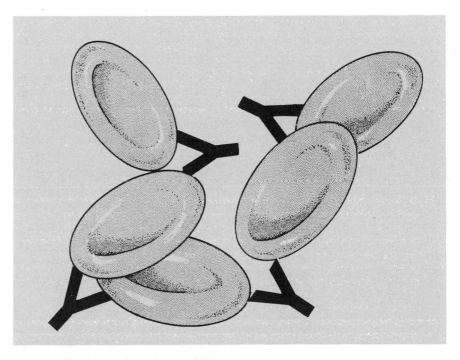

Figure 1.6I Under conditions in which the distance between the cells has been reduced, agglutination of red cells by IgG antibodies may take place without the addition of anti-human serum.

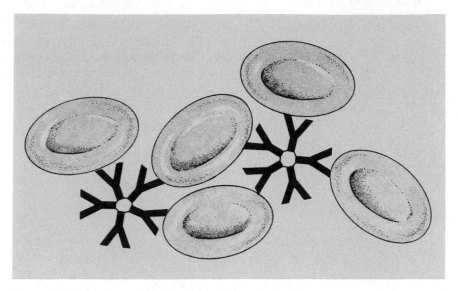

Figure 1.6J Agglutination of red cells by IgM antibodies does not require alteration of intercellular distance because the antibody molecule is large enough to bridge the distance between cells suspended in saline.

One of the factors in the formula for calculating zeta potential is the dielectric constant of the medium. This is one of the most easily controlled factors. If the dielectric constant is raised, the zeta potential is lowered. Solutions containing dipolar molecules, such as bovine albumin, raise the dielectric constant. Adding albumin to the antibody/red cell mixture potentiates agglutination by increasing the dielectric constant of the suspending medium, lowering the zeta potential and thus reducing the minimum distance between the cells.

The second proposed explanation of red blood cell agglutination by antibody is the water-of-hydration theory, which states that cells in solution are kept apart by water molecules tightly bound to the cell surface. The water molecules further away from the cell become less and less tightly bound until they are free to move in the suspending medium. Antibodies which bind to the cells decrease this water-of-hydration layer and thus increase the ability of the cell to agglutinate. (About 40 molecules of water are displaced for every antibody molecule bound to the cell.) Charged polymers also disturb the bound water molecules and thus enhance aggregation of the red cells.

It was stated earlier that the force of repulsion between cells can be reduced in two ways — first, by altering the medium in which the cells are suspended during testing, and second, by directly reducing the negative charge of the red cell. Much of the negative charge is contributed by the sialic acid residues that are a part of **glycophorin A**, the glycoprotein that carries M and N blood group antigens. **Proteolytic enzymes** such as trypsin, papain, ficin and bromelin break certain peptide bonds of proteins. Trypsin is the most specific in its action. It cleaves polypeptide chains at the sites of both arginine and lysine, while other proteolytic enzymes cleave somewhat indiscriminately. As a result of the enzyme treatment, the ends of the proteins with the attached oligosaccharides (sialic acid) are lost from the cell. In this way, enzymes reduce the net negative charge of red cells, but this is only one of the effects of enzymes. The M and N antigens are lost when red cells are enzyme-treated, and other antigens may also be altered, weakened or lost, depending on the particular enzyme used. Those antigens sometimes involved are S, s and Fy^a. In contrast, enzyme treatment of cells enhances some antigen-antibody reactions. Removal of the terminal portion of proteins with the attached oligosaccharide molecules alters the surface structure so that other antigens are now more accessible to their antibodies. The Rh antibodies are uniformly more reactive with enzyme-treated cells. This may be due, at least in part, to removal of protruding chains that interfere with the Rh antibody's ability to reach the Rh antigens which are, presumably, closer to the cell membrane.

In contrast to the action of proteolytic enzymes, neuraminidase treatment of red cells removes only sialic acid residues, leaving the protein chains intact. Removal of sialic acid results in the loss of M and N antigen receptors, but does not enhance the reaction of the cell with Rh antibodies.

1.6 QUESTIONS

Red blood cells which simply have antibodies attached to them (without any visible changes in the cells) are called

sensitized

_____ cells.

Cells which have been sensitized by incomplete antibodies can be

anti-human serum

agglutinated *in vitro* using _____,
which contains antibodies to human gamma globulins.

When antigen-antibody reactions lead to red blood cell lysis, the lysis is mediated by the:

☐ coagulation system.

complement system.

☐ complement system.

Red blood cell lysis is caused by the components of the complement system which attach to the red cell:

☐ early in the sequence.

late in the sequence.

☐ late in the sequence.

When only some of the components of the complement sequence are fixed to red blood cells, lysis may not occur. However, these complement-sensitized cells can be agglutinated *in vitro* using anti-

complement

human serum specific for _____.

Anti-human serum specific for IgG antibodies is produced by injecting rabbits with purified human:

☐ alpha globulin.

☐ gamma globulin.

gamma globulin.

☐ beta globulin.

Anti-human serum specific for complement is produced by injecting rabbits with purified human:

☐ alpha globulin.

beta globulin.

☐ beta globulin.

☐ gamma globulin.

Any test which incorporates anti-human serum is called a(n)

antiglobulin

_____ test.

Match the following:

1   A

1 _____ direct Coombs test

A anti-human serum is added to agglutinate the patient's sensitized cells

2   B

2 _____ indirect Coombs test

B reagent cells are added to be sensitized by antibodies in the patient's serum

If unattached globulins are not removed during the washing phase of the antiglobulin test, a false

☐ positive

negative

☐ negative

test may result.

Match the following:

1   A

1 _____ IgG antibodies

A agglutination of red blood cells requires anti-human serum or altering the suspending medium

2   B

2 _____ IgM antibodies

B agglutination of red blood cells proceeds without adding anti-human serum

The surface of a red blood cell has a strong net:

negative charge.

☐ negative charge.

☐ positive charge.

This net surface charge of red blood cells is maintained by the large number of

☐ A or B antigens

☐ protein antigens

sialic acid residues

☐ sialic acid residues

attached to the cell membrane.

The minimum distance between two red cells is influenced by

the _____ potential.

By raising the dielectric constant of the medium, the zeta potential is:

☐ raised.

☐ lowered.

Antibodies which bind to red cells

☐ decrease

☐ increase

the water-of-hydration of the cells.

Proteolytic enzymes such as trypsin decrease the net negative charge
of a red cell by:

☐ adding positive charges to the cell's surface.

☐ cleaving negative charges from the cell's surface.

Match the following:

1 ____ M and N

2 ____ Rh

A antibodies are more reactive
with enzyme-treated red cells

B antigens are lost when cells
are treated with proteolytic
enzymes

Match the following:

1 ____ trypsin

2 ____ neuraminidase

A breaks polypeptide bonds

B releases sialic acid

Chapter Two:

Blood Group Genetics

Objectives for Chapter Two

Upon completion of this chapter you should be able to:

2.1 • Describe the basic genetic concepts which are relevant to blood group systems

2.2 • Explain how genes effect the production of blood group antigens

2.3 • Define the following terms:
  • allele
  • homozygous
  • heterozygous
  • dosage effect
  • amorph
  • structural gene
  • regulator gene
  • genotype
  • phenotype

2.4 • List the four ABO blood groups and their corresponding antigens and expected antibodies

  • Identify the structures of the A and B antigens and describe how they are synthesized from a common precursor chain

2.5 • Identify the structure of the P_1 antigen and describe how it is synthesized from the same precursor as the A and B antigens

2.6 • Describe the functions of the *Le* gene and the *Se* gene in the synthesis of Le^a and Le^b antigens

  • Define sialoglycoprotein

2.7 • Describe the major genetic concepts of the MNSs system

2.8 • Compare and contrast the Fisher-Race and Wiener theories of inheritance of the Rh system

  • Explain why the D antigen is called a mosaic antigen and the importance of this in Rh blood typing

  • Describe gene interaction and its importance within the Rh system

2.9 • Describe the minus-minus phenotypes of the ABO, Rh, Kell, Duffy, Kidd and Lutheran systems

2.1

What is the relevance of blood group genetics?

It would be natural to ask why a knowledge of genetics is important to the operation of a blood bank or a transfusion service. First, some knowledge of the genetic control of antigens is necessary when seeking an explanation for unexpected reactions observed in the laboratory and especially when suggesting additional testing to resolve the problem. Second, there is certainly no question that anyone doing parentage testing must have a very substantial knowledge of the genetics of blood groups. Perhaps most important, the subject is fascinating, challenging and can be a stimulating aspect of a very critical health care function that may otherwise seem routine.

It is possible to postulate mechanisms of genetic control of an antigen only if the chemical structure of the antigen is known. The antigenic determinants of the ABO, P, Lewis and MN systems are oligosaccharides and the structure of the major antigens in each system is well established. Consequently, more is known of their genetic control than of most other blood group systems. While it is known that Rh antigens are primarily protein, their structures are poorly understood and little is known of their genetic control. Information about the chemical structure of the antigens of other systems is not sufficient to allow more than the postulation of simple theories to explain their origins.

It is not the purpose of this book to discuss genetics in great detail. A level of understanding summarized in the following facts is assumed:

- Humans have 22 pairs of **autosomes** and a pair of **sex chromosomes** (XX in females and XY in males).

- **Chromosomes** are made up of **deoxyribonucleic acid (DNA)** — which carries the genetic message — and proteins whose functions are not altogether clear.

- During the reduction division stage of meiosis, homologous chromosomes exchange segments of genetic material so that each chromosome entering the gamete contains variable amounts of maternal and paternal genetic material. This process of exchanging segments of chromosomes is called **crossing over**.

- A new organism is formed when an ovum and a sperm, each carrying one-half of the genetic material, unite to form a **zygote**. This union re-establishes the normal complement of chromosomes.

- In each body cell most genes are "turned off" or inactive. The process by which they are "turned on" is not completely understood.

- The building blocks of DNA are called **nucleotides**, each of which is composed of a phosphate group, deoxyribose and a nitrogenous base. The phosphate group and deoxyribose are the same in all nucleotides but there are four different nitrogenous bases — two purines (adenine and guanine) and two pyrimidines (cytosine and thymine). The genetic message is determined by the sequence in which these nucleotides are joined.

- DNA serves as a template to produce **messenger ribonucleic acid (mRNA)** and the genetic message is transcribed to the mRNA. The message is made up of three-letter words called **codons**, the letters being the nucleotides. Each codon designates one amino acid.

- Messenger RNA moves into the **cytoplasm** and is "read" by the **ribosomes**. The amino acids are organized into proper sequences for specific proteins according to the instructions imparted to the ribosomes by the mRNA. If one of the nucleotides is altered by **mutation** or if the nucleotides are rearranged within the codon, the new sequence is read by the ribosome and a different amino acid is formed. An entirely new protein may be the result.

- Amino acids which are joined by peptide bonds are called **polypeptides**. Polypeptides are the basis for all proteins.

2.1 QUESTIONS

The antigenic determinants of the ABO, P, Lewis and MN systems are:

☐ lipoproteins.

☐ oligosaccharides.

Humans have _____ pair(s) of autosomes and

_____ pair(s) of sex chromosomes.

Human chromosomes are composed of

☐ DNA

☐ RNA

and proteins.

Each ovum or sperm contains

☐ one-quarter

☐ one-half

☐ a full set

of the genetic material of the zygote to be formed.

Paired chromosomes exchange genetic material in a process called:

☐ nondisjunction.

☐ crossing over.

An ovum and a sperm unite to form a:

☐ zygote.

☐ gamete.

Most of the genetic material in a mature, differentiated body cell is:

☐ "turned on."

☐ "turned off."

---

oligosaccharides.

22

one

DNA

one-half

crossing over.

zygote.

"turned off."

61

Answer Column

1 B

2 A

1 A

2 B

the sequence of nucleotides in the DNA.

messenger ribonucleic acid (mRNA)

three

ribosomes

completely altered.

Match the following:

1 _____ the building blocks of DNA   A   amino acids

2 _____ the building blocks of proteins   B   nucleotides

Match the following:

1 _____ adenine and guanine   A   purines

2 _____ cytosine and thymine   B   pyrimidines

The genetic message is determined by:

☐ the length of DNA strands.

☐ the sequence of nucleotides in the DNA.

DNA serves as the template for the synthesis of

_____ .

In the genetic code, each codon consists of

☐ two

☐ three

☐ four

nucleotides.

Messenger RNA is "read" by _____
which are in the cytoplasm.

If a mutation or rearrangement of the nucleotides in DNA occurs, the protein for which that segment of DNA codes may be:

☐ completely altered.

☐ corrected by extracellular processing.

amino acids

Polypeptides consist of

☐ amino acids

☐ oligosaccharides

joined by peptide bonds.

2.2

How do genes determine blood group antigens?

It is probable that those blood group antigens which are proteins are the direct product of gene action. The polypeptide may be inserted into the membrane as a single chain or it may be folded, perhaps joined to other chains, and inserted as a complex structure. On the other hand, because genes control the production of proteins only, the construction of oligosaccharide antigens must involve an intermediate step. This intermediate step is the production of enzymes (which are proteins) called **transferases** which assemble individual sugars into chains and more complex molecules. Transferases catalyze the transfer of a particular sugar molecule from its source to a specific receptor molecule (substrate). As each transferase adds its sugar, a new structure is formed and this structure may then be the substrate used by another transferase. The mechanism of transferase action is illustrated in Figure 2.2A.

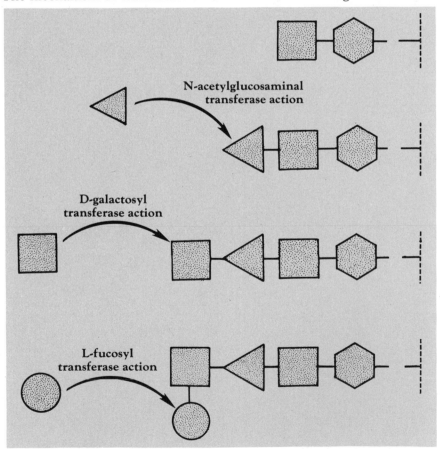

Figure 2.2A Schematic illustration of the action of transferases. Each transferase adds a sugar molecule to the growing oligosaccharide chain. The substrate for each transferase is the product of the previous transferase-catalyzed reaction. The symbols represent the following sugars: hexagon – N-acetylgalactosamine; square – D-galactose; triangle – N-acetylglucosamine; circle – L-fucose.

1	A
2	B
transferases	
1	A
2	B

2.2 QUESTIONS

Match the following:

1 ____ protein antigens   A   direct products of gene action

2 ____ oligosaccharides   B   require an intermediate step

Enzymes which assemble sugars into oligosaccharide chains are called

_____ .

Match the following:

1 ____ catalyst   A   enzyme

2 ____ receptor molecule   B   substrate

2.3

How do genes interact?

Alternative genes, any one of which may occupy a given locus on a chromosome, are called **allelomorphs**, **allelic genes** or simply **alleles**. Most blood group systems have two (or occasionally three) major alleles. A system in which two or more alleles are commonly found is said to be **polymorphic**. Regardless of the number of allelic genes possible at a gene locus, only one can occupy each locus on a given chromosome. Since chromosomes are inherited in pairs, one from each parent, blood group genes also occur in pairs. When the two loci of paired chromosomes are occupied by identical genes, the person is said to be **homozygous** for that gene, and the antigen it controls is produced in **double dose**. When the two loci are occupied by different alleles, the person is said to be **heterozygous** and each antigen is produced in **single dose**. Homozygous and heterozygous inheritance is illustrated in Figure 2.3A. It should be stressed here that the expression of a gene (genetic trait) may be dominant or recessive to the trait expressed by its allele. In blood groups most genes are codominant in expression; that is, the gene trait or antigen is demonstrated regardless of whether the gene is paired with an unlike allele (heterozygous) or whether both of the paired genes are the same (homozygous).

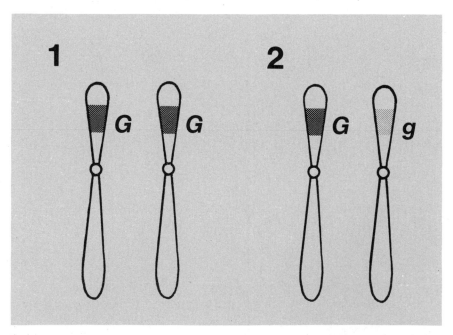

Figure 2.3A Illustration of homozygous vs. heterozygous inheritance. G and g are two alleles for the same locus. The individual in (1) is homozygous for G; i.e., both chromosomes carry the G gene. The individual in (2) is heterozygous; i.e., the pair of chromosomes carries different genes, G and g.

At least in theory, a cell which contains two like genes should produce twice as much antigen as a heterozygote; however, the difference in quantity of antigen on the red cell as a result of the expression of one gene or two genes may not always be demonstrable in routine laboratory tests. In some procedures and especially in some blood group systems, this variable expression of antigen strength is observable and is referred to as the **dosage effect**. It can be useful in antibody identification using reagent red cells of known genotypes. For example, the serum of a patient with anti-c often shows dosage by reacting more strongly with homozygous cells (*c/c*) than with heterozygous cells (*C/c*). Recognition of dosage can also be a useful tool when selected antisera are used to establish the probable genotype of family members with rare blood groups, especially when silent genes are involved. (When the product of a gene cannot be detected by any currently available techniques, the gene is referred to as a **silent gene** or an **amorph**.)

The genes which direct the construction of proteins are called **structural genes**. The synthesis of both protein antigens and oligosaccharide antigens is often further complicated by the necessity of the prior action of other structural genes, the presence of amorphic genes and the presence of regulator genes. The necessity of prior action of other structural genes is best understood if related to oligosaccharide antigens. As was shown in Figure 2.2A, the ability of a transferase to assemble its antigen is dependent on the presence of a **substrate**. If the substrate is not present, the transferase cannot construct its antigen. The substrate is itself the product of a structural gene. Amorphic genes can be the alleles of functioning genes, as is true of *h*, *se* and *le* in the pairs *H/h*, *Se/se* and *Le/le*. On the other hand they can be the third allele of a pair of structural genes. Nearly every blood group system illustrates this concept, e.g., $Fy^a/Fy^b/Fy$ where Fy is an amorph. Regulator genes further complicate the synthesis of antigens. By definition, products of regulator genes control the rate at which the products of other genes are synthesized. In blood group genetics there is evidence of a variety of regulator genes, but their products have not been identified. Therefore the mechanism of their action is not fully understood. For this reason they have been called **regulators, modifiers** or **inhibitors** in different systems. Throughout this book the term ''modifier'' is used most often.

Before proceeding to a discussion of each blood group system, it is necessary to understand two additional terms: phenotype and genotype. The **phenotype** of a person is the description of observed traits or the results of tests, e.g., blue eyes, long legs or blood group A. The **genotype** is the genetic constitution which produces the traits. Since it is not possible to probe into the genetic makeup of a person in any direct way, the genotype must be deduced. Since any deduction is an interpretation of observations, it is subject to error. For this reason a genotype must always be expressed as a ''probable'' genotype.

2.3 QUESTIONS

When one of several genes can occupy a given chromosomal locus, the genes are called _____ _____ .

allelomorphs, allelic genes or alleles

Blood group systems most commonly have

☐ two (or occasionally three)

☐ always three or more

☐ usually four or more

major alleles.

two (or occasionally three)

When a blood group system has two or more alleles, the system is called _____ .

polymorphic

Like chromosomes, blood group genes are inherited:

☐ singly.

☐ in pairs.

in pairs.

When identical genes are present at paired chromosomal loci, the person is said to be _____ .

homozygous

When two different genes are present, one at each of the pair of chromosomal loci, the person is said to be _____ .

heterozygous

Match the following:

1 ____ homozygous   A antigens produced in a single dose

2 ____ heterozygous   B antigens produced in double dose

1 B

2 A

The terms "dominant" and "recessive" refer to:

☐ genes themselves.

☐ gene expression (genetic traits).

gene expression (genetic traits).

codominant.

When the allelic genes of paired loci differ and both are expressed, gene expression is said to be:

☐ dominant.

☐ codominant.

The expression of most blood group genes is:

☐ dominant.

☐ recessive.

codominant.

☐ codominant.

When the difference between heterozygous and homozygous gene expression is observable in routine laboratory tests, this difference is referred to as:

☐ allele imbalance.

dosage effect.

☐ dosage effect.

When currently available techniques are unable to detect the product

silent; amorphic

of a gene, the gene is called a _____ or _____ gene.

Match the following:

1 B

1 ___ structural gene   A   may direct the synthesis of a molecule which regulates the rate of synthesis of another gene product

2 A

2 ___ regulator gene   B   directs the synthesis of proteins

Match the following:

1 A

1 ___ phenotype   A   observed trait or test result

2 B

2 ___ genotype   B   genetic makeup

2.4

What are the major genetic concepts of the ABO system?

In the ABO system there are three major alleles — A, B and O — any one of which may occupy the ABO locus on each of the paired chromosomes. The ABO locus has been shown to be on chromosome number nine. The O gene does not produce any demonstrable red cell antigen, thus it is an amorph. As shown in Table 2.4A, people are classified phenotypically as A, B, AB or O but phenotype A may result from the genotype AA or AO and likewise for the phenotype B.

Table 2.4A The relationship between ABO phenotypes and genotypes.

Phenotype	Genotype
A	AA AO
B	BB BO
AB	AB
O	OO

As stated before, the A and B antigens are primarily oligosaccharides constructed by gene-specified transferases. The A and B antigens are schematically illustrated in Figure 2.4B. The antigenic determinant is the single terminal sugar of a large oligosaccharide chain but its ability to react with antibody is also dependent on the arrangement of the few sugars close to the site of attachment. The determinant for the A antigen is N-acetylgalactosamine and for the B antigen, D-galactose. The A and B gene-specified transferases add their specific sugars to an oligosaccharide chain called the H chain. The H chain must first be created by the action of the H gene-specified transferase which adds its specific sugar (fucose) to an oligosaccharide known as the **precursor chain**.

Precursor chains are of two types which differ from each other only in the carbon-to-carbon linkage between the terminal galactose and the subterminal N-acetylglucosamine. The chains found as an integral part of the red blood cell membrane are predominantly type II chains while those in body fluids are type I. Type I and type II precursor chains are illustrated in Figure 2.4C.

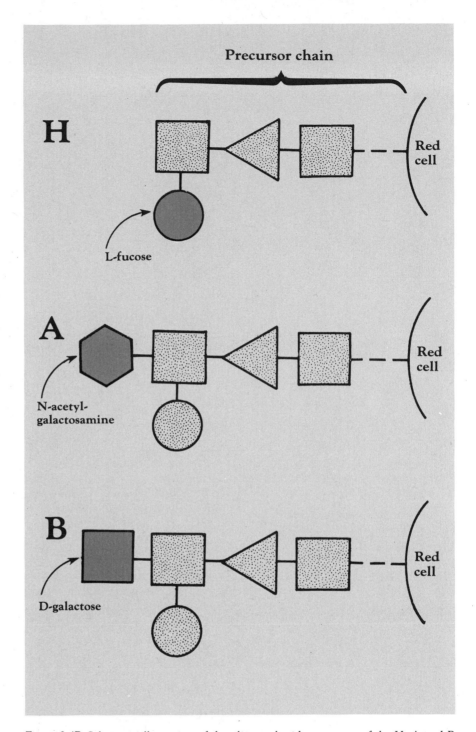

Figure 2.4B Schematic illustration of the oligosaccharide structures of the H, A and B antigens. The precursor chain is the substrate for the H gene-specified fucosyl transferase; the H chain is the substrate for both A and B gene-specified transferases, which add N-acetylgalactosamine and D-galactose, respectively, to the H chain. In the AB individual N-acetylgalactosamine and D-galactose are added to different chains of the same red cell. The symbols represent the following sugars: hexagon – N-acetylgalactosamine; square – D-galactose; triangle – N-acetylglucosamine; circle – L-fucose. The broken line represents additional sugars.

1 Type I Chain

D-galactose — **N-acetylglucosamine** — **D-galactose**

Type I 1-3 linkage

2 Type II Chain

D-galactose — **N-acetylglucosamine** — **D-galactose**

Type II 1-4 linkage

Figure 2.4C (1) An illustration of the terminal sugars of a type I precursor chain with 1-3 carbon-to-carbon linkage between the terminal D-galactose and N-acetylglucosamine. (2) A type II chain with 1-4 linkage between the same sugars. In Figure 2.4B, a square represents D-galactose and a triangle represents N-acetylglucosamine.

Because there is no A or B gene-specified transferase in group O individuals to convert the H chains to A or B, group O cells retain a large amount of H antigen (unconverted H chain). As the conversion from H antigen to A and/or B antigens takes place in group A, B and AB individuals, the H antigenic determinant is masked by the A and/or B sugars; therefore, A, B and AB red cells have little exposed H antigen and react weakly, if at all, with anti-H.

The *H* gene and its allele *h* are inherited independently of the allelic A, B and O genes. The *H* gene is expressed in both the homozygous (*H/H*) and the heterozygous (*H/h*) state; the *h* gene is an amorph. When no *H* gene is inherited (*h/h*) — an extremely rare occurrence — no H chains can be created, so the A and B transferases have no substrate to which to add their sugars. Thus the rare *h/h* individual appears to be group O even though he or she may have A and/or B genes which produce normal transferases. The phenotype of *h/h* individuals is commonly called **Bombay** for the city in which the discovery was made; it is more properly described as O_h or ABH_{null}.

People who have inherited variants of *A* and *B* genes are occasionally encountered. They are usually recognized by the fact that the variant gene produces a weaker than normal red cell antigen — in some cases because of a difference in the transferase produced. Different levels of expression of A or B on red cells are classified into subgroups. About 80 percent of group A individuals are A_1 and the remaining 20 percent are A_2. It has been shown that the transferase produced by the A_2 gene differs from that produced by A_1 in that it is less efficient in converting H chains to A; however, the terminal sugar of A_2 is the same as the terminal sugar of A_1. The difference between the A_1 and A_2 phenotypes is illustrated in Figure 2.4D. Other subgroups of A are rare and each is the result of a different genetic background. Subgroups of B are rarely encountered.

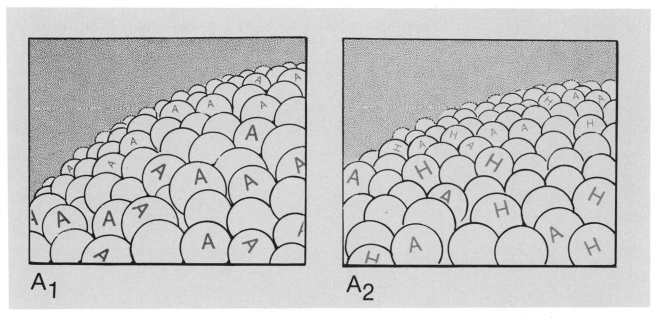

Figure 2.4D Illustration of the A_1 and A_2 phenotypes. In the A_1 individual, the N-acetylgalactosaminal transferase efficiently converts H antigens to A antigens. In contrast, the A_2 individual has fewer A antigens and more residual H antigens due to the inheritance of a less efficient N-acetylgalactosaminal transferase.

Normally, blood group antigens are stable throughout life, but they may be altered as a result of disease. Antigens previously demonstrated on the red cells of a patient may no longer be detectable, or the cells may acquire a pseudoantigen. Transferase levels and activity play a major role in the loss and acquisition of red cell antigens in health as well as in disease. These altered antigens will be discussed in more detail in Chapter Three.

As discussed previously, A, B and H antigens are not confined to red cells but may be present in body fluids also. The secretion of A, B and H **substances** in saliva and other fluids is controlled by a pair of alleles, *Se* and *se*, called **secretor genes**. Secretion of A, B and H soluble substances is accomplished even when only one locus carries *Se*. There can be no *Se* when *se* is present on both chromosomes. The gene *se* is an amorph. The locus occupied by the secretor genes is not linked to the ABO locus. This is to say that the genes at each of the loci are inherited independently. (See Focus Question 2.6 for a further explanation of the role of the *Se* gene.) Persons who have A, B and/or H substances in saliva are called **secretors** and the following will be present in their saliva:

Blood Group	Substances in Saliva
A	A and H
B	B and H
AB	A, B and H
O	H

Provided the person is a secretor (whether *Se/Se* or *Se/se*), saliva tests can be helpful in defining a subgroup or in resolving the genetic makeup of an individual who appears to have an unusual blood group. About 80 percent of Caucasians are secretors.

2.4 QUESTIONS

The ABO blood group system has _____ major alleles.

The ABO locus is on chromosome number:

☐ one.

☐ six.

☐ nine.

Since the O gene does not produce any demonstrable red cell antigen, it is considered a(n):

☐ modifier gene.

☐ amorph.

Match the following ABO phenotypes with the appropriate genotypes:

1 ____ group A		A	AA
2 ____ group B		B	BB
3 ____ group O		C	OO
4 ____ group AB		D	AO
		E	BO
		F	AB

The antigenic determinant of an A, B or H antigen is the

_____

_____ .

Match the following antigenic determinants with the appropriate antigen:

1 ____ H antigen		A	L-fucose
2 ____ B antigen		B	D-galactose

Type I and type II precursor chains differ in:

☐ their terminal sugars.

☐ the carbon-to-carbon linkage between their terminal and subterminal sugars.

Match the following:

1 ____ type I precursor chain

2 ____ type II precursor chain

A found in body fluids

B an integral part of the red cell membrane

Which ABO blood group reacts most strongly with anti-H?

_____

Of the A, B, O and H genes, which are allelic and which gene is independent of the other(s)?

allelic _____

independent _____

Match the following:

1 ____ H gene

2 ____ h gene

A L-fucosyl transferase

B no gene product detectable

No H chains are synthesized when a person is:

☐ H/h

☐ h/h

A and B antigens

☐ are

☐ are not

synthesized in the rare h/h individual.

Homozygous *h/h* individuals appear to be group:

☐ A

☐ B

☐ O

Phenotypic names for *h/h* individuals are

_____, _____,

and _____.

A_1 and A_2 differ in:

☐ the efficiency with which their transferases convert H chains to A chains.

☐ the carbon-to-carbon linkage between the terminal and subterminal sugars in the oligosaccharide chain.

Blood group antigens are normally stable throughout life but they

may be altered by _____.

The *Se* and *se* genes control the secretion of A, B and H

_____

in body fluids such as saliva.

The locus for secretor genes is:

☐ linked to the ABO locus.

☐ not linked to the ABO locus.

List the substances found in the saliva of secretors for each of the ABO blood groups:

group A _____

group B _____

group O _____

group AB _____

O

Bombay, O$_h$, ABH$_{null}$

the efficiency with which their transferases convert H chains to A chains.

disease

substances

not linked to the ABO locus.

A and H

B and H

H

A, B and H

Se/Se

Se/se

80

Which of the following genotypes would produce phenotypic secretors?

☐ Se/Se

☐ Se/se

☐ se/se

Approximately what percentage of Caucasians are secretors?

☐ 50

☐ 80

2.5

What are the major genetic concepts of the P system?

The P system is like the ABO system in that the antigens are primarily oligosaccharide chains constructed by transferases. Whereas the antigens have been characterized, the sequence of transferase activity is not completely resolved. Since the genetic control of the transferases is not known, the system must be described in terms of phenotypes and antigens.

There are two major phenotypes — P_1 and P_2. The designation P_2 is used to indicate the absence of P_1; there is no P_2 antigen. As can be seen in Figure 2.5A, the P_1 antigen is constructed by adding D-galactose to the type II precursor chain of the red cell membrane. In the P system this precursor is called **paragloboside**, even though it is the same substrate used by the H gene-specified transferase to form **type II H chains.**

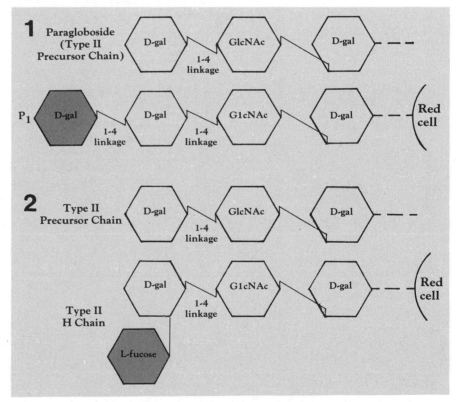

Figure 2.5A (1) The type II precursor chain (called paragloboside when discussing the P system) is the substrate not only for the transferase that makes the P_1 antigen but also (2) for the H gene-specified fucosyl transferase that makes type II H chains. In order to illustrate the importance of carbon-to-carbon linkage, the shapes of the individual sugars of the oligosaccharide chains are all represented as hexagons and designated by names. The three terminal sugars of the chain are shown; the dotted line represents the remaining sugars which are not specifically illustrated. GlcNAc is the short symbol for N-acetylglucosamine.

The P system is further complicated by the presence of another oligosaccharide chain similar to paragloboside, called **globoside**. The globoside structure forms the antigen P which is common to P_1 and P_2 phenotypes. As can be seen in Figure 2.5B, the production of P appears to be independent of P_1; however, globoside and paragloboside may result from some of the same transferases. For this reason, when a single transferase is altered, changes may take place in both globoside and paragloboside. In very rare persons, the transferase that completes globoside is missing and this incomplete chain forms the antigen of the P^k phenotype. P^k can be found with either P_1 or P_2 but, because of the interaction within the system, the P_1 antigen is very weak in the person who has the phenotype P_1^k, i.e., has both P_1 and P^k. Another very rare phenotype called pp or Tj(a–) has no P_1, P or P^k antigens.

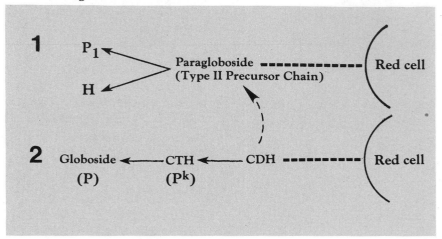

Figure 2.5B In the figure, arrows represent transferases that add specific sugars to form new antigens. (1) Paragloboside is the substrate for either P_1 or H gene-specified transferases, as was shown graphically in Figure 2.5A. (2) CDH (ceramide dihexoside — a two-sugar chain) is the substrate needed to form P^k, and CTH (ceramide trihexoside — a three-sugar chain) is the substrate needed to form P. The interaction between the two oligosaccharides is not completely understood, as is indicated by the broken arrow.

2.5 QUESTIONS

P_1 antigens are:

☐ proteins.

☐ oligosaccharides.

Like A and B antigens, P_1 antigens are synthesized by:

☐ ribosomes.

☐ transferases.

P_1 antigens and H antigens are synthesized from

☐ the same

☐ a different

precursor chain.

The type II precursor chain in the ABO system is the same structure as

☐ paragloboside

☐ globoside

in the P system.

The P_1 antigen is formed by the addition of

☐ L-fucose

☐ D-galactose

to paragloboside.

The P_1 antigen is not synthesized when its transferase is absent and the resulting phenotype is called:

☐ P_2

☐ pp

When the antigens P_1, P and P^k are absent the phenotype is called

_____ .

---

oligosaccharides.

transferases.

the same

paragloboside

D-galactose

P_2

pp or Tj(a−)

2.6

What are the major genetic concepts of the Lewis system?

Lewis antigens detected on red blood cells by the usual blood grouping techniques are not an integral part of the red cells; they are adsorbed from the plasma. The antigens are primarily oligosaccharides and their structures are well defined. The genetic control of their synthesis is also understood. The concepts are not difficult if certain principles which have been discussed before are accepted.

- Oligosaccharide antigens are constructed by transferases.

- Each specific sugar is added to a precise substrate. This pairing is determined by the genetic code controlling the transferase.

- Transferases can produce antigen only if the proper substrate has been preformed.

- Some transferases can use more than one substrate.

- When a new sugar is added to a substrate, a new antigen may be formed which masks the antigen formed by the previous structure.

Two pairs of allelic genes produce transferases which function in concert to produce Lewis antigens: the Lewis genes, *Le* and *le*, and the secretor genes, *Se* and *se*. Both *le* and *se* are amorphs. As is shown in Figure 2.6A, the Le gene-specified transferase can use either of two substrates — the type I precursor chain or the **type I H chain**. When the *Le* gene is inherited but the *Se* gene is not, one fucose molecule is added to the subterminal sugar of the type I precursor chain creating Le^a soluble antigen. When the *Le* gene and the *Se* gene are both present, the *Se* gene adds a fucose to the precursor chain, creating a type I H chain. Following this, the *Le* gene can add a fucose to this type I H chain. This structure is the soluble Le^b antigen.

As has just been discussed, either Le^a or Le^b soluble plasma antigens are constructed by the interaction of *Le* and *Se*. The Lewis red cell phenotype results from adsorption of one or the other. When no *Le* is inherited, no soluble Lewis substances are formed and the red cell phenotype is Le(a–b–). Table 2.6B shows the red cell phenotypes which result from the inheritance of different combinations of *Le*, *le*, *Se* and *se*.

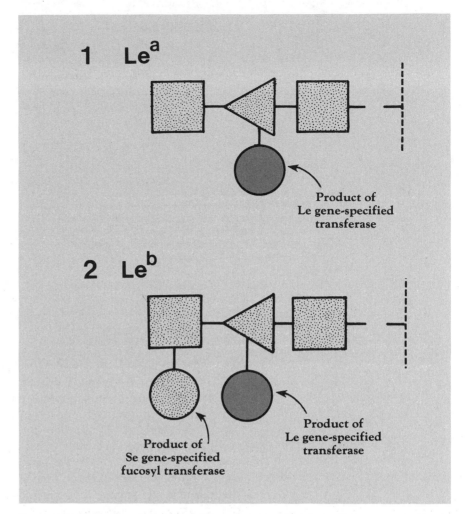

Figure 2.6A Schematic illustration of the structures of the Le^a and Le^b antigens. The *Le* gene can add fucose to either of two substrates — the type I precursor chain to make Le^a or the type I H chain to make Le^b. (1) If the individual is *se/se*, the Le^a antigen is formed by the addition of L-fucose to the type I precursor chain. (2) If the individual has inherited an *Se* gene, the type I precursor chain is converted by the action of the Se gene-specified fucosyl transferase to an H chain and the further action of *Le* creates the Le^b antigen. Symbols represent the following sugars: square – D-galactose; triangle – N-acetylglucosamine; circle – L-fucose.

The Le^a soluble antigen is not a substrate for any gene-specified transferase, but Le^b is a substrate for A and B transferases. In A, B and AB persons much of the Le^b structure is masked by further action of A and/or B gene-specified transferases. The antigen that results is called ALe^b or BLe^b and when absorbed by the red cell, little Le^b antigen is available to react with anti-Le^b. This explains the poor reaction of group A or group B red cells with human anti-Le^b sera.

Table 2.6B Derivation of Lewis red cell phenotypes. (1) Nonsecretors of ABH (*se/se*) who inherit *Le* have the red cell phenotype Le(a+b−). (2) Secretors of ABH who inherit *Le* have the red cell phenotype Le(a−b+). Regardless of the inheritance of *Se*, if no *Le* is inherited (*le/le*), the red cell phenotype is Le(a−b−).

		Le/Le or *Le/le*	*le/le*
1	NONSECRETORS *se/se*	Le(a+b−)	Le(a−b−)
2	SECRETORS *Se/Se* or *Se/se*	Le(a−b+)	Le(a−b−)

The Primary Role of the *Se* Gene

It has been known for many years that the ability to secrete ABH substances in body fluids depends on a pair of allelic genes, *Se* and *se*. The gene *Se* functions when present on one or both paired loci. The mechanism by which this is accomplished has only recently been elucidated. As has been discussed earlier in this focus question, the *Se* gene controls the production of the **fucosyl transferase** that adds fucose to the type I precursor chain and thus constructs the type I H chain. In this context the *Se* gene is sometimes designated H(*Se*). A person of the genotype *se/se* cannot secrete A, B or H substances because the lack of the Se gene-specified fucosyl transferase precludes construction of type I H chains in body fluids. In contrast, the *H* gene produces a similar fucosyl transferase but the H gene-specified fucosyl transferase uses the type II precursor chain of the red cell as a substrate. Failure to produce H chains on red cells results in the Bombay phenotype.

In summary, evidence suggests that *Se* and *H* are two distinct genes which code for different fucosyl transferases, one using type I chains as a substrate and the other using type II chains. By accepting this concept and extending it further, it is possible to clarify the terms **Bombay** and **para-Bombay**. Persons who lack *H* (*h/h*) and who lack *Se* (*se/se*) have no type II H chains on their red cells and have no type I H chains in their body fluids. These persons have the classic Bombay or ABH$_{null}$ phenotype. But some persons, called para-Bombays, lack H on their red cells but have H in their secretions. These people have no *H* gene and no type II H chains on their cells but have *Se* (*Se/Se* or *Se/se*) and therefore make type I H chains in body fluids. Depending on which A and B genes are inherited, para-Bombays will secrete A and/or B substances as well as H. It has been proposed that the terms Bombay-secretor and Bombay-nonsecretor be used instead of para-Bombay and Bombay.

2.6 QUESTIONS

Match the following:

1 A

2 B

1 _____ ABH antigens	A	synthesized by red cells
2 _____ Lewis antigens	B	adsorbed from the plasma

Lewis antigens are:

☐ proteins.

oligosaccharides. ☐ oligosaccharides.

Lewis antigens are constructed by enzymes called

transferases _____ .

substrate Each transferase adds a sugar to a precise _____
which must have already been formed.

Which of the following is true?

☐ Each transferase can use only one substrate.

Some transferases can use ☐ Some transferases can use more than one substrate.
more than one substrate.

The addition of a new sugar to a substrate may produce a new:

☐ peptide.

antigen. ☐ antigen.

For the following Lewis red cell phenotypes, state whether the *Le* and
Se genes are present or absent:

	Le gene	*Se* gene
present; absent Le(a+b−)	_____	_____
present; present Le(a−b+)	_____	_____

For the following Lewis red cell phenotypes, state which Lewis antigen is present on red cells:

Le(a+b−) _____

Le(a−b+) _____

Match the following:

1 ____ Le^a A   one fucose molecule added to the type I precursor chain

2 ____ Le^b B   one fucose molecule added to the type I H chain

A and B transferases of the ABO system will add sugars to which Lewis substance(s)?

☐ Le^a

☐ Le^b

☐ both

The *Se* gene controls the production of a fucosyl transferase which adds fucose to the

☐ type I

☐ type II

precursor chain.

Which gene controls the production of a fucosyl transferase which adds fucose to a type II precursor chain?

_____

Match the following:

1 ____ Bombay   A   *h/h* and *se/se*

2 ____ para-Bombay   B   *h/h* and *Se/Se* or
                            h/h and *Se/se*

Answer column (left margin):

Le^a

Le^b

1 A

2 B

Le^b

type I

H gene

1 A

2 B

2.7

What are the major genetic concepts of the MNSs system?

With the exception of ABO and Lewis, probably more is known of the chemical structure of the antigens of the MNSs system than any other system, but controversy over the explanation of the genetic control has become heated from time to time. The structures that carry MNS and s antigens are glycoproteins; that is, they are composed of polypeptide chains to which sugars have been added. Because the majority of the sugars are sialic acid, the more correct terminology is **sialoglycoprotein (SGP)**.

It is generally accepted that the antigenic determinants of the system are the oligosaccharides, but the configuration of these sugars is controlled by the sequence of the amino acid residues to which they are attached. The sequence of amino acids is determined by the M and N genes. That the antigenic determinants are solely oligosaccharides has been challenged; there is some evidence that the amino acids may also be a part of the antigenic determinants. The following facts are established:

- Allelic genes M and N control the transmission of M and N antigens to the next generation.

- Another pair of alleles, S and s, controls the transmission of S and s antigens to the next generation.

- The Ss locus appears to be contiguous with the locus for MN.

- Because of the close linkage, M or N and S or s are almost always transmitted as a unit. (In decreasing frequency the sequence is Ns, Ms, MS and NS.)

- Two of the glycoproteins which protrude from the cell membrane, as was shown in Figure 1.1D, carry the MNSs antigens. One (**glycophorin A**) carries the antigenic determinants of M and N. The other (**glycophorin B**) carries S and s.

- The precise amino acid sequence of the polypeptide chains of glycophorin A has been determined. Glycophorin A (MN SGP) occurs in two forms which differ from each other in the first and fifth amino acid residues of the segment of the chain external to the cell, depending on whether the blood group gene M or N has been inherited. The differences in the amino acid residues of M and N are shown in Figure 2.7A.

- The amino acid sequence of the terminal portion of glycophorin B (Ss SGP) is identical to the amino acid sequence of the glycophorin A that results from an *N* gene, but the attached sugar structures differ from the N antigen.

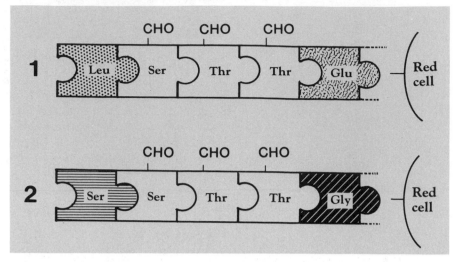

Figure 2.7A The amino acid sequence of the glycophorin A (MN SGP) when the structural gene is *N* is shown in (1). When the genetic control is M, the amino acid sequence is as shown in (2). The heterozygous M/N person makes both structures. Abbreviations for amino acids: Leu – leucine; Ser – serine; Thr – threonine; Glu – glutamic acid; Gly – glycine; CHO – alkali-labile oligosaccharide (composed primarily of sialic acid).

Very rarely, antigens of the MNSs system are weakened or missing. This condition can be due either to abnormal polypeptide chains or to altered oligosaccharides.

As stated, the locus for M and N is very closely linked to the locus for S and s. Only a few families have been found that confirm crossing over between the two loci. Often the coupling within a family, as is illustrated in Figure 2.7B, can be shown by testing for all four antigens.

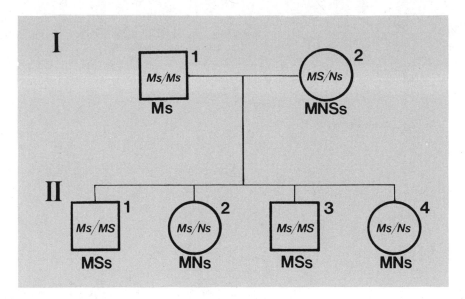

Figure 2.7B This family tree illustrates the close linkage of the *MN* locus with the *Ss* locus. Phenotypes are shown below the symbols. Judging from his phenotype, the genotype of the father (I-1) can only be *Ms/Ms*. Each child has inherited *Ms* from the father. The children who inherited M from their mother (I-2) also inherited S, while those who inherited N received *s*. Therefore, the pairing (coupling) in this mother is *MS* and *Ns*.

sialoglycoproteins.

2.7 QUESTIONS

The antigens of the MNSs blood group are:

☐ glycolipids.

☐ sialoglycoproteins.

Match the following antigenic determinants with the appropriate cell-surface proteins:

1 _____ S and s   A   glycophorin A

2 _____ M and N   B   glycophorin B

Depending upon whether the blood group is M or N, glycophorin A differs in the

☐ first

☐ fifth

☐ first and fifth

amino acid(s) of the external segment.

The terminal amino acid segment of glycophorin B is the same as that of glycophorin A when the blood group is:

☐ M

☐ N

The configuration of the oligosaccharides in the MNSs system is controlled by the:

☐ *Se* gene.

☐ sequence of the amino acid residues.

The loci for M and N and for S and s are:

☐ independently inherited.

☐ closely linked.

Margin answers (left column):

sialoglycoproteins.

1 B

2 A

first and fifth

N

sequence of the amino acid residues.

closely linked.

2.8

What are the major genetic concepts of the Rh system?

Because knowledge of the molecular structure of the Rh antigens is minimal, any proposed schema of genetic control must be recognized as theoretical. However, certain assumptions have been useful in providing a basis for determining the probability of inheriting genes of the Rh system.

Nomenclature

A primary purpose for studying the theories of inheritance is to better understand the notations used in the Rh system, especially when postulating the probable genotype of an individual. In the years since the Fisher-Race and Wiener theories of Rh inheritance were proposed, much has been learned about genetics as well as the Rh system. Neither of the two original theories can accommodate all the facts now known, but parts of both can be incorporated into current concepts.

According to the **Fisher-Race theory**, the antigens of the Rh system are determined by three pairs of genes which occupy closely-linked loci. In the Rh system there are usually only two or three alleles at each locus. As shown in Figure 2.8A, one locus is occupied by either *D* or *d*; another by *C, c* or *C^w*; and a third is occupied by *E* or *e*. According to the Fisher-Race concept, the gene *d* appears to be a silent gene or an amorph because there is no demonstrable product of *d*. The gene *d* is assumed to be present when *D* is absent. The order of the loci is thought to be D-C-E.

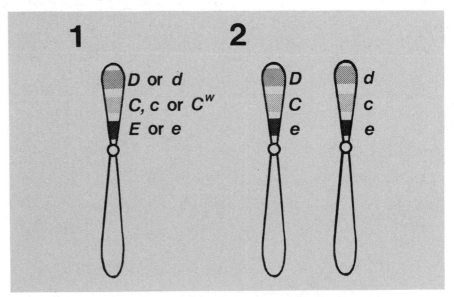

Figure 2.8A (1) Illustration of the Fisher-Race theory of three closely linked loci and their possible alleles. (2) Illustration of a *DCe/dce* individual.

The three loci that carry the Rh genes are so closely linked on the chromosome that they never separate but are passed from generation to generation as a unit or gene complex. An offspring of the *DCe/dce* individual illustrated in Figure 2.8A will inherit either *DCe* or *dce* from the parent, but not a combination such as *dCe*. Should such a combination occur, it indicates crossing over. This has never been proven to occur in the Rh system of man, although one family is reported which can be interpreted as a possible example of either crossing over or mutation.

In the Fisher-Race notation, the gene and the red cell antigen it produces are given the same symbol; however, the letter is italicized when referring to the gene. With the exception of the amorph *d*, each of the allelic genes mentioned so far controls the presence of its respective antigen on the red cells. As can be seen in Figure 2.8B, the gene complex *DCe* determines the presence of antigens D, C and e on the red cells. If the same gene complex were on both of the paired chromosomes, D, C and e would be the only Rh antigens demonstrable on the cells. However, if one chromosome carried *DCe* and the other *DcE*, the antigens present would be D, C, c, E and e. Each antigen (except d) is recognizable by testing the red cells with a specific antiserum.

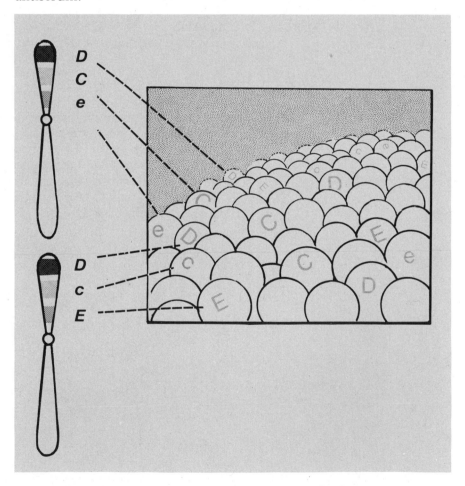

Figure 2.8B Illustration of antigen production according to the Fisher-Race concept.

In contrast, the **Wiener theory** postulates that two genes, one on each chromosome of the pair, control the entire expression of the Rh system in one individual. The genes at the two loci may be alike (homozygous) or different from each other (heterozygous). Multiple alleles of this gene exist. As shown in Figure 2.8C, the eight major alleles are called R^0, R^1, R^2, R^z, r, r', r'' and r^y.

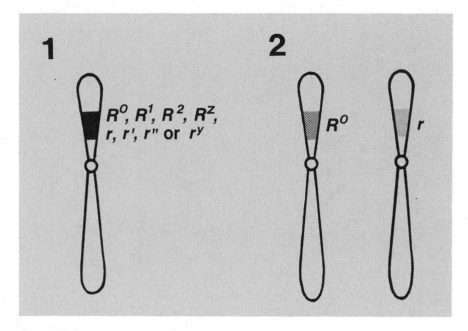

Figure 2.8C Illustration of the Wiener hypothesis of a single gene locus and the possible alleles at that locus. (2) Illustration of an R^0/r individual.

According to Wiener's hypothesis, each gene produces a structure on the red cell called an **agglutinogen**, and each agglutinogen can be identified by its parts or **factors** that react with specific antibodies. As illustrated in Figure 2.8D the gene R^1 has been inherited on one chromosome and the gene r at the same locus on the other chromosome. The gene R^1 determines the agglutinogen Rh_1 on the red cell and this agglutinogen is made up of at least three factors — $\mathbf{Rh_o}$, **rh′** and **hr″**. The gene r determines the agglutinogen rh on the red cell distinguished by its factors **hr′** and **hr″**.

These two theories are the basis for two notations currently in use for the Rh system. Table 2.8E compares Fisher-Race and Wiener notations.

Both the Fisher-Race and Wiener notations are based on genetic concepts or theories of inheritance, while Rosenfield and his co-workers proposed a notation based on results of tests. Each of the various Rh antisera is assigned an arbitrary number. The **Rosenfield system** permits an unbiased phenotype determination based solely on the results observed with the antisera employed. A partial list of the numbers assigned is given in Table 2.8F. The phenotype of a given cell is expressed by the base symbol Rh followed by a colon and a list of the numbers of the specific Rh antisera employed. Each number is separated by a comma, and a minus sign precedes the number if a negative result was obtained with that particular antiserum. For example, a cell of the phenotype Rh: 1, 2, –3, 4 has been tested with only four antisera. The antiserum designated number 3 (anti-E) failed to react, while antisera numbers l, 2 and 4 (anti-D, anti-C and anti-c, respectively) reacted with the cell.

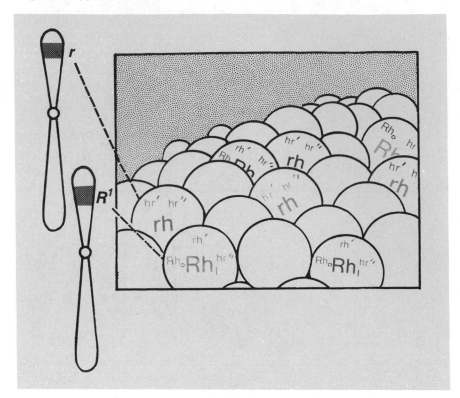

Figure 2.8D Illustration of antigen production in the Wiener system. Note that the R^1 gene directs the production of the Rh_1 agglutinogen, which is made up of at least three factors ($\mathbf{Rh_o}$, $\mathbf{rh'}$ and $\mathbf{hr''}$), while the r gene directs the production of the rh agglutinogen, which is made up of two factors ($\mathbf{hr'}$ and $\mathbf{hr''}$).

Table 2.8E Comparison of the Fisher-Race and Wiener notations for the Rh system.

Fisher-Race Notation		Wiener Notation		
Gene Complex	Antigens	Genes	Agglutinogens	Factors
Dce	D, c, e	R^o	Rh_o	$\mathbf{Rh_o, hr', hr''}$
DCe	D, C, e	R^1	Rh_1	$\mathbf{Rh_o, rh', hr''}$
DcE	D, c, E	R^2	Rh_2	$\mathbf{Rh_o, hr', rh''}$
DCE	D, C, E	R^z	Rh_z	$\mathbf{Rh_o, rh', rh''}$
dce	c, e	r	rh	$\mathbf{hr', hr''}$
dCe	C, e	r'	rh'	$\mathbf{rh', hr''}$
dcE	c, E	r''	rh''	$\mathbf{hr', rh''}$
dCE	C, E	r^y	rh_y	$\mathbf{rh', rh''}$

Table 2.8F Numerical notation as suggested by Rosenfield.

Antigenic Determinant			Corresponding Antibody	
Rosenfield	Wiener	Fisher-Race		
Rh 1	Rh_o	D	Anti-Rh 1	Anti-D
Rh 2	rh'	C	Anti-Rh 2	Anti-C
Rh 3	rh"	E	Anti-Rh 3	Anti-E
Rh 4	hr'	c	Anti-Rh 4	Anti-c
Rh 5	hr"	e	Anti-Rh 5	Anti-e
Rh 6	hr	ce(f)	Anti-Rh 6	Anti-f
Rh 7	rh	Ce	Anti-Rh 7	Anti-Ce
Rh 8	rh^{w1}	C^w	Anti-Rh 8	Anti-C^w
Rh 10	hr^v	$V(ce^s)$	Anti-Rh 10	Anti-V
Rh 12	rh^G	G	Anti-Rh 12	Anti-G
Rh 19	hr^s	—	Anti-Rh 19	Anti-hr^s
Rh 20	—	VS	Anti-Rh 20	Anti-VS

Genotyping

The major determination to be made in Rh typing is to distinguish which bloods are **Rh positive** and which are **Rh negative**. The term "Rh positive" refers only to the presence of D antigen or its variant D^u on the red cells; it does not indicate whether both or only one of the chromosomes carry the D gene. The presumptive genotype can be determined for any individual and this determination is useful in parentage studies or to predict the probability that the husband of an Rh negative woman is heterozygous or homozygous for D. The Rh negative woman cannot contribute D to any of her offspring. If her husband is homozygous so that both loci are occupied by D, all their children will inherit one of his D genes and be D positive. On the other hand, if the father is heterozygous and only one chromosome carries D, then only those children inheriting D (statistically, one-half of them) will be D positive. The other half will not inherit D from the father (or the mother) and will be D (Rh_o) negative. This inheritance is illustrated in Figure 2.8G.

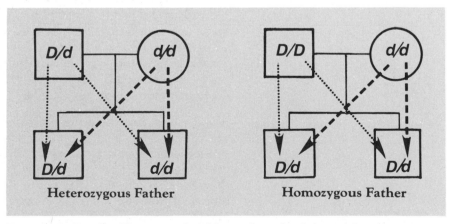

Figure 2.8G Possible Rh types of children when the father is heterozygous or homozygous.

Since there is no "anti-d," genotyping cannot be done by simply testing red cells for D and d antigens. Instead, advantage is taken of statistical probability in the relationship of D with C, c, E and e. The molecular structure which carries Rh antigens is complex and, in addition to D, may also carry C or c and E or e. Therefore five Rh antisera are used to determine the antigens present on (or absent from) the red cells, and the probable genotype is ascertained by reference to a chart. The frequency of each genotype was determined by tests of large numbers of Caucasoid persons and their families. As is shown in Table 2.8H, the results obtained in the laboratory are matched with those on the chart. From among the genotypes that would react in the same way as the cells being tested, the genotype with the highest frequency is selected as the most probable.

Table 2.8H Presumptive genotypes based on reactions with five antisera.

Reactions with Anti- D C E c e	Probable genotype		% Freq.	Second most likely genotype		% Freq.
+ + o + +	DCe/dce	R^1r	32.7	DCe/Dce	R^1R^o	2.2
+ + o o +	DCe/DCe	R^1R^1	17.7	DCe/dCe	R^1r'	0.8
+ + + + +	DCe/DcE	R^1R^2	12.0	DCe/dcE or DcE/dCe	R^1r'' R^2r'	1.0 0.3
+ o + + +	DcE/dce	R^2r	11.0	DcE/Dce	R^2R^o	0.7
+ o + + o	DcE/DcE	R^2R^2	2.0	DcE/dcE	R^2r''	0.3
+ o o + +	Dce/dce	R^or	2.0	Dce/Dce	R^oR^o	0.1
o o o + +	dce/dce	rr	15.0			
o + o + +	dCe/dce	r'r	0.8			
o o + + +	dcE/dce	r''r	0.9			

In the first example of Table 2.8H, tests indicate that the red cells carry the antigens D, C, c and e, but not E. The corresponding genes controlling these antigens must be present on the chromosomes of the person, but how they are grouped is not known. The antigens on the red cells could be the result of two possibilities: DCe on one chromosome and dce on the other, or DCe on one and Dce on the other. These genotypes are written as DCe/dce for the former and DCe/Dce for the latter. Since 32.7 percent of Caucasians are DCe/dce while only 2.2 percent are DCe/Dce, it follows that the assignment of the more common genotype (DCe/dce) is more probably correct.

It is essential that the genotype of a person be listed as "presumptive" or "most probable" since, in almost every instance, a second or third genotype is possible based on the results obtained in tests for the red cell antigens. Tests of the red cells of the parents and/or children of the person in question may confirm the genotype or clarify the possibilities. Otherwise, we must depend on the statistical evidence that one is more common than the others and is therefore more likely to be the correct assumption.

Every racial group varies to some extent from those listed here. Even within small countries the frequency of certain antigens will vary slightly from one area to another. Among American Blacks the most common gene complex is *Dce*. To allow for this increase, *DCe*, *DcE* and *dce* are all less common than in Caucasians.

Gene Complex	% in Caucasians	% in Blacks
Dce	2	46
DCe	40	16
DcE	14	9
dce	38	25

The Structure of Rh Antigens

Whereas there are many antigens or antigenic determinants within the Rh system, it is now believed that they are each part of a unit carried on one of the protein molecules embedded in the red cell membrane. Many copies of this molecule are present on each cell. Rh antigens have not been found in soluble form and it is difficult to isolate proteins from the red cell membrane in a purified form. Although extensive analysis of the Rh antigen has not been accomplished, certain facts are known.

Depending on the procedure used to do the analysis, the molecular weight of the protein carrying D (and probably all Rh antigens) has been determined to be from 170,000 to 300,000 daltons. The individual antigenic determinants may be much smaller. This size will have more meaning if it is compared with the size of an antibody. IgG molecules have a molecular weight of about 150,000 daltons, not greatly different from the weight of the molecule that carries the antigenic determinants. Even if only a small portion of the protein protrudes from the surface of the cell membrane, it is sufficient for antigen-antibody interaction since only a small portion of the antibody molecule constitutes the antigen-binding site.

The internal structure of the molecule is not known but presumably it is like other proteins in that the sequence of amino acid residues in the primary chain controls the final configuration of the molecule. There is little question that groups of Rh antigens are inherited *en bloc*. The most common of these groups are DCe, DcE and ce. (There is no d antigen.) Whether these antigens are the product of one gene which controls the construction of the protein molecule or more than one gene is still not known. It seems quite probable, however, that there is more than one gene, that these genes are contiguous on the chromosome, and are in an area that rarely (if ever) is subject to crossing over. A set of contiguous genes inherited as a unit is called a **gene complex**. A gene complex codes for a specific polypeptide chain that may be folded and perhaps attached to other polypeptide chains; the result is a protein of a characteristic shape. Since the sequence of amino acids in the primary chain is under genetic control, the configuration of the molecule will vary from one person to another depending on the genes he or she inherits. A person inheriting the gene complex *DCe* will have one structure exposed on the cell surface, while a person with the gene complex *DcE* will have a slightly different structure. It is not known whether the Rh antigen is totally protein. If there are oligosaccharide components of the antigen, these could also enter into the surface conformation and contribute to the enormous complexity of the molecule.

This genetic explanation for the structure of antigens can be extended to take into account the differences among single antigenic determinants. For example, C and E may differ in only one amino acid substitution which may have been caused by the mutation or transposition of a single nucleotide in the DNA. This small change in the primary structure may alter the configuration of the molecule, thereby creating a new antigenic determinant.

The term "D^u" has been used to designate some weakly reactive Rh positive cells. The majority of cells which type as Rh positive but are of the weakly reacting variety D^u are probably quantitatively deficient in D antigen; however, the structure of the antigen may not be qualitatively different from D. This reduction in the number of antigenic sites on the red cells is genetically controlled, as can be seen in family studies. The majority of cells which are labeled Rh positive, D^u variant, are of this quantitatively deficient type.

As shown in Figure 2.8I, the D antigen, whether from a D positive or D^u positive individual, is considered to be a mosaic of many parts or many antigenic determinants, called **epitopes**. Under certain circumstances, perhaps by mutation or unequal crossing over, one or more of these epitopes is missing or changed, or a substitution has occurred, so that the shape of the total D antigen is altered. Presumably this change involves a very small portion of the D antigen. Since most of the antigen remains intact and most Rh antisera are **heterogeneous**, the red cells still type as Rh positive. In some instances there are greater changes and these cells react only in the test for D^u. If the person lacking an epitope were to receive common D positive cells, either by pregnancy or transfusion, that epitope of the total antigen may be recognized as foreign by the recipient and an antibody may be produced against that epitope only. Although this antibody is directed to only one epitope of the total antigen, it would react with all common Rh positive cells because they have the total antigen. It is not known how many epitopes there are to the mosaic. Based on the work of Tippett in England and work done in the Philip Levine Laboratories, no fewer than eight variants of D and D^u have been identified. Some variants may be the result of more than one missing epitope. In the Philip Levine Laboratories, "mosaic" D positive people (identified by the fact that they produced anti-D) could be divided into about 40 percent who were clearly D positive and 60 percent who were Rh positive, D^u variant.

It is not difficult to fit the mosaic concept of D and D^u into the schema of genetic control discussed on the previous pages. The locus occupied by the *D* gene may be highly mutable and each mutation may produce a small variation in the primary amino acid chain. Some of these changes are so small that the final configuration is not easily distinguished from the common D antigen. Others cause greater dif-

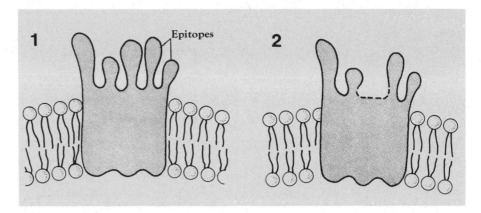

Figure 2.8I (1) Illustration of the normal D antigen which is made up of several epitopes. (2) Illustration of an altered D antigen in which one of the epitopes is missing. An individual with altered D antigens would type as D positive but if exposed to D positive cells, could produce antibodies to the epitope present on the normal D antigen but missing from the altered D antigen. The antibody would behave like anti-D.

ferences, but the altered antigens still resemble the common D antigen in their ability to cause the production of anti-D in an Rh negative person. Other changes result in more significant differences, but these altered antigens can be recognized as Rh positive, provided the anti-D reagent used is made from pools of serum from a large number of donors. Such pools contribute a heterogeneous population of antibodies, some of which will react with different epitopes of the Rh molecule.

As discussed above, some red cells of the D^u phenotype have a reduced number of Rh antigens on their surface; some (or all) of these may also be mosaic D^u, but the research required to determine how many are quantitatively different, how many are mosaics, and how many may be both has not been done.

Occasionally, red cells appear to be D^u but, when testing the family, it becomes evident that the trait is not inherited from either parent. The cells of this type of D^u are usually of the genotype DCe/dCe. It has been suggested that the C gene in *trans* position (i.e., on the opposite chromosome) suppresses the expression of D on the red cells. This is an example of one gene or gene product interacting with another on the partner chromosome to produce an effect which is not evident when the chromosomes segregate in the next generation. The effects of such gene interaction are illustrated in Figure 2.8J. When DCe is freed of the influence of dCe, there is no longer any suppression of D. There is a wide variation in the degree of suppression in different families, and rarely is it of such magnitude that it will be noticed in testing with commercial anti-D sera. Cells with this type of suppressed D, called gene-interaction D^u, are much less common than the hereditary D^u produced by genes which code either for fewer D antigen sites or for an altered D antigen.

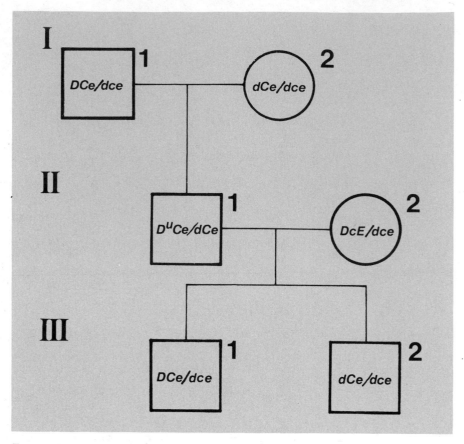

Figure 2.8J Suppression of the expression of *D* gene by *C* gene on the opposite chromosome (II-1). When the *D* gene is freed of the influence of the *C* gene in *trans* position as in III-1, there is no longer any suppression of *D*.

There is another cause for weakened Rh antigens. Genes which are not part of the Rh system and are inherited independently can interact to modify the expression of the Rh structural genes. These modifier (or regulator) genes can totally suppress the structural Rh genes. The result is the Rh_{null} phenotype. When tested with any or all Rh antisera, the cells which are Rh_{null} fail to react; they appear to be devoid of Rh antigens. However, the Rh genes are normal as shown by the fact that Rh_{null} individuals transmit to their offspring functional Rh genes which they inherited from their parents. This is illustrated in Figure 2.8K. The terminology assigned to this modifier gene, which Levine postulated to explain the Rh_{null} phenotype, is X^0r. Most people have the common allele X^1r which does not suppress Rh. When X^0r is heterozygous (X^0r/X^1r), partial suppression results; when the gene is homozygous (X^0r/X^0r), there is essentially complete suppression of the Rh genes.

Another modifier gene postulated by Chown and called X^Q may be a mutant form of X^0r. Partial suppression of the Rh antigens was shown in a Canadian family. The propositus was clearly *DCe/DcE* (R^1R^2) but each antigen was considerably weaker than normal.

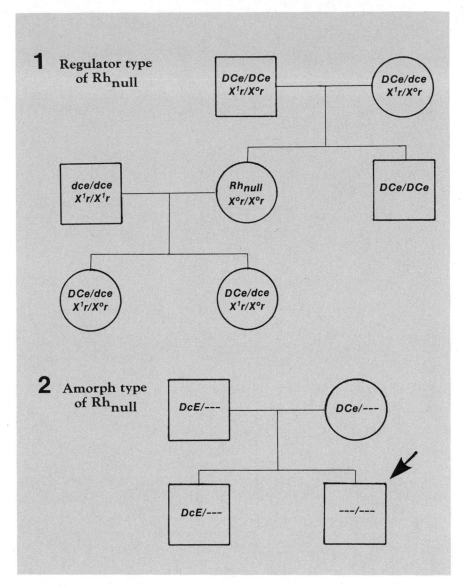

1 Regulator type of Rh_{null}

2 Amorph type of Rh_{null}

Figure 2.8K Types of Rh$_{null}$. (1) In the regulator type of Rh$_{null}$ the regulator genes $X^o r/X^o r$ suppress the Rh structural genes. In the heterozygote $X^1 r/X^o r$, Rh antigens are present on red cells but may be weak. (2) In the amorph type of Rh$_{null}$ no Rh antigens can be detected on the red cells. The heterozygote expresses the genes of one chromosome; for example, $DcE/---$ expresses D, c and E but no C or e. This phenotype could be erroneously interpreted as the probable genotype DcE/DcE.

2.8 QUESTIONS

The molecular structures of the Rh antigens are understood in:

☐ considerable detail.

☐ minimal detail.

All the facts currently known about the Rh system can be accounted for by:

☐ the Fisher-Race theory of inheritance.

☐ the Wiener theory of inheritance.

☐ neither theory

Match the following:

1 ___ Fisher-Race theory   A   one pair of genes

2 ___ Wiener theory   B   three pairs of closely linked genes

For each of the loci as proposed in the Fisher-Race theory, list the possible alleles:

D locus _____

C locus _____

E locus _____

In the Fisher-Race theory which allele is thought to be a silent gene?

_____

According to the Fisher-Race theory, which antigens could be determined in the laboratory in a person whose genotype was DCe/dCE?

_____

In the Wiener theory,

☐ five

☐ seven

☐ eight

major alleles are postulated as possible occupants of the Rh locus.

---

minimal detail.

neither theory

1   B

2   A

D, d

C, c, C^w

E, e

d

D, C, E and e

eight

According to the Wiener theory, each allele controls the synthesis of a structure on the red cell membrane called a(n) _____ which can be identified by its parts or _____ that react with specific antibodies.

In contrast to the Fisher-Race and the Wiener nomenclature, the Rosenfield nomenclature is based on:

☐ genetic concepts.

☐ antisera test results.

The terms "Rh positive" and "Rh negative" refer to the presence or absence of the antigen _____ .

If a woman is Rh negative and her husband is heterozygous for D, then the probability that a child of theirs will inherit D is:

☐ 25 percent.

☐ 50 percent.

☐ 75 percent.

Postulating a genotype in the Rh system is done by:

☐ testing with antisera to D, C, c, E and e antigens.

☐ statistical methods based on testing with antisera to D, C, c, E and e antigens.

Rh genotypes are considered "presumptive" or "most probable" because there are alternative choices in:

☐ almost every instance.

☐ very few instances.

The frequency of Rh genotypes

☐ is the same

☐ differs

in different racial groups.

The antigenic determinants of the Rh system are now believed to be

☐ part of a single unit

☐ separate units

embedded in the red cell membrane.

The antigenic determinant of the D antigen is probably a relatively

☐ small

☐ large

portion of the protein carrying the Rh antigens.

A set of contiguous genes inherited as a unit is called a(n)

_____ .

Small changes in the amino acid sequence may give rise to

_____ on the red cell surface.

Weakly reactive D positive cells are designated:

☐ D^w

☐ D^u

The D antigen is thought to be made up of many antigenic determinants called:

☐ allotopes.

☐ epitopes.

Anti-D specific for one epitope could be produced by a person missing an epitope if the person were exposed to:

☐ common D positive red cells.

☐ red cells missing the same epitope.

The C gene in

☐ *trans*

☐ *cis*

position may suppress the expression of *D* on red cells.

Match the following conditions with the appropriate label (each label may be used more than once):

1 _____ a decreased number of normal D antigens

A   gene interaction D^u

2 _____ suppression of Rh genes by independently inherited genes

B   hereditary D^u

3 _____ an abnormally structured D antigen (missing or altered epitopes)

C Rh_{null}

4 _____ suppression of a D gene by a C gene in *trans* position

2.9

What are the major genetic concepts of other blood group systems?

Whereas the chemical structure of all blood group antigens may not be known, some observations are common to most systems, and certain genetic concepts offer a logical explanation for the observations. Among these are the following:

- In most systems the antigens are controlled by two (or occasionally three) alleles, and there are **minus-minus (null) phenotypes** in which neither of the alleles is expressed.

- In at least two systems (Kell and Lutheran) there are many pairs of allelic genes within a single gene complex.

Minus-Minus Phenotype

In nearly every system, including ABO and Rh, there is a null or minus-minus phenotype: group O, O_h, Rh_{null}, Fy(a–b–), Jk(a–b–), Lu(a–b–). With few exceptions, these null phenotypes can arise from either of two types of genetic control. A minus-minus phenotype may be the result of either an amorphic (silent) gene which occupies both loci of the paired chromosomes, or a regulator or modifier gene located some distance away, which suppresses the action of the structural blood group genes. The former is referred to as the recessive type of minus-minus phenotype, meaning that the amorph must be homozygous to completely block antigen production. The latter type may be either (1) a dominant trait in which the regulator gene suppresses the blood group gene even when only one regulator gene is inherited, or (2) a recessive trait in which the regulator gene must be present at both paired loci (homozygous) in order to suppress the production of antigen.

In other words, the minus-minus phenotypes are the result of either **amorphic blood group genes** which are always recessive in effect or **modifier genes** — not linked to the genes whose expression they modify — which may be either dominant or recessive in effect.

Several important aspects of these two genetic concepts — amorphs and modifiers — must be emphasized. An amorphic gene produces no demonstrable antigen; however, if it occupies the locus on only one of the pair of chromosomes, the other gene functions normally. To produce the minus-minus phenotype, both loci must be occupied by the silent gene. In contrast, modifiers influence both genes of the pair, but their effect varies considerably and they rarely suppress antigen production totally. This incomplete suppression can be illustrated by the fact that antibody can be adsorbed to and eluted from minus-minus phenotypes of the modifier type in each system, but not from the minus-minus phenotypes that result from amorphic genes. It should also be noted that modifier genes can affect more than one blood group system. The modifier gene $In(Lu)$ of the Lutheran system also modifies the antigens of the P system. These two genetic concepts will be discussed relative to the major blood group systems in the remainder of this focus question.

As was discussed following Focus Question 2.4, the amorph O of the ABO system fails to make any blood group antigen. The presence of the gene is difficult to recognize except when homozygous. Tracing the inheritance of A and B genes in certain families may reveal obligate heterozygotes, that is, A/O or B/O. The H gene is necessary for the production of the substrate for the A and/or B gene-specified transferases but is not genetically part of the ABO system. When it is replaced on both chromosomes by its allele h, no H, A or B antigens can be expressed on red cells. The resulting phenotype is called O_h or ABH_{null}.

In the Rh system the effect of either amorphs or modifying genes can be observed as Rh_{null} cells. Rh_{null} cells carry none of the numerous Rh antigens. The amorph (---) is difficult to recognize except when homozygous. Although a very rare occurrence, the presence of an amorph must be considered when test results in family studies do not conform to expected patterns. For example, the genotype $DCe/---$ will appear to be of the probable genotype DCe/DCe because no c or E antigen is demonstrable. In contrast to amorphs, the modifying gene called $X^o r$ is not part of the Rh gene complex. When the $X^o r$ gene is homozygous, none of the genes of the Rh complex are expressed; the fact that the Rh genes function normally when transmitted to the next generation indicates the Rh genes are normal but are prevented from functioning. The regulator type of Rh_{null} is more common than the amorphic type although both are extremely rare.

In the Kell system there is evidence of a modifier gene X^k which appears to function much like $X^l r$ of the Rh system. When X^k is absent, there is little or no expression of Kell system antigens. The null phenotype of the Kell system can also result from the amorphic gene K^o. None of the many Kell system antigens is expressed on the red cells of a K^o/K^o individual. In the heterozygous condition, K^o is difficult to recognize; the red cells of a person with the genotype k/K^o type as K negative and k positive, as do 90 percent of the random population. The possibility that the gene K^o is causing part of the discrepant results should be considered if one finds an abnormal inheritance pattern within the Kell system.

Minus-minus phenotypes of the Duffy system also may have two genetic backgrounds. Because the amorph Fy is common in Blacks, phenotypes of the Duffy system are difficult to translate into genotypes, as can be seen in the following chart.

Phenotypes	Most Probable Genotypes	
	Caucasians	Blacks
Fy(a–b+)	Fy^b/Fy^b	Fy^b/Fy
Fy(a+b–)	Fy^a/Fy^a	Fy^a/Fy
Fy(a+b+)	Fy^a/Fy^b	Fy^a/Fy^b
Fy(a–b–)	Very rare	Fy/Fy

The existence of a modifier gene affecting the Duffy system has been postulated to explain the very rare Fy(a–b–) phenotype of Caucasians.

In the Kidd system the null phenotype appears to be derived from a modifying gene. Evidence for a silent Jk gene is lacking. The Jk(a–b–) phenotype is very rare in Caucasians but more common in Polynesians and some Orientals.

In the Lutheran system the effects of either an amorph Lu or a modifier gene $In(Lu)$ may explain the Lu(a–b–) phenotype in different families. The term In(Lu) is derived from "inhibitor of Lutheran." Although the amorphic Lu(a–b–) phenotype exists, it is extremely rare.

The second genetic concept pertinent to understanding blood groups (mentioned in the beginning of Focus Question 2.9) is that of multiple paired allelic genes or **gene clusters**. The concept was discussed in relation to the Rh system in which the loci for D, C and E are closely linked, but the term "gene cluster" was not introduced at that time. In the Rh system the term "gene complex" is more often used. Both terms designate groups of paired loci so closely linked that crossing over is rarely, if ever, observed. Numerous gene pairs are clustered in both the Kell and Lutheran systems. In these clusters the genes function individually, although they often interact to weaken certain antigens expressed by other genes within the cluster. For example, in the Rh system D is not expressed as fully in the presence of C (DCe) as it is in the presence of E (DcE). In the Kell system Kp^a when paired with K^o has a suppressive effect on the other genes of the cluster.

The null phenotype of each system involves the entire gene cluster. In the Rh system the modifier X^or, when homozygous, suppresses the entire Rh gene cluster of both chromosomes. The mechanism by which this is accomplished is not known. The modifier in the Kell system, called X^k (located on the X chromosome), apparently controls the production of whatever precursor is needed for the action of the Kell structural gene cluster of both chromosomes. In the Lutheran system $In(Lu)$ is an autosomal dominant modifier that, even in the heterozygous state, does not allow the expression of any of the structural Lutheran genes. In the Rh, Kell and Lutheran systems, the amorphs designated –––, K^o and Lu, respectively, also affect all the numerous structural genes of the cluster. However, in contrast to a modifier gene which affects the gene cluster on both chromosomes, an amorph affects the gene cluster of one chromosome only. Therefore, it is only in very rare instances where the amorph is homozygous that both chromosomes are non-functioning and no antigen is produced. In Figure 2.9A, the Kell system is used to illustrate the concept of gene clusters and amorphs.

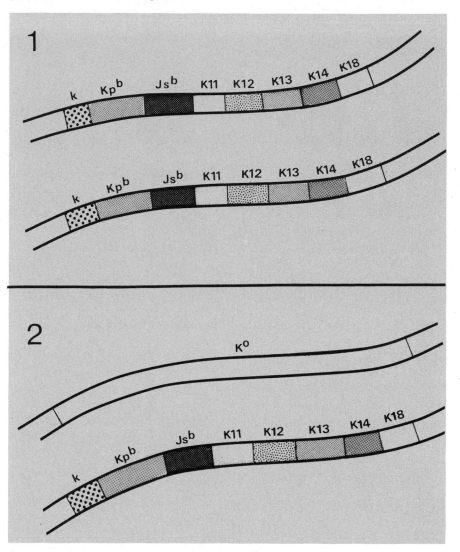

Figure 2.9A An illustration of the Kell gene cluster and the effect of amorphic genes. The cluster illustrated in (1) is the most common genotype. Most people are homozygous for the Kell genes shown in the cluster. The rare K^o paired with the common gene cluster is shown in (2). Note that when the chromosome carries the amorph, all genes of the cluster are replaced by the amorph. The other gene of the pair functions normally and the red cell phenotype is usually not distinguishable from the normal homozygote shown in (1) except by family studies.

Xg^a was the first blood group antigen known to be controlled by a gene on the X chromosome. Because the loci of many non-blood group genes are known to be on the X chromosome, the prospect of tracing them through generations and predicting their inheritance based on blood group tests was very exciting. However, Xg^a has proven to be somewhat of a disappointment to immunohematologists. The gene locus for Xg^a is too far from any other recognized loci to measure, and no meaningful linkage data with disease-related genes have been established.

2.9 QUESTIONS

homozygous amorph.

A minus-minus phenotype may be the result of a:

☐ homozygous amorph.

☐ single amorph.

Such a minus-minus phenotype is called a:

recessive minus-minus
phenotype.

☐ recessive minus-minus phenotype.

☐ dominant minus-minus phenotype.

A minus-minus phenotype may also be the result of a modifier gene

structural blood group
genes

which suppresses the action of _____ .

Match the following:

1   A

2   B

1 ____ homozygous amorph   A   no antigen detectable

2 ____ modifier   B   a small amount of antigen
detectable

Which type of gene can affect more than one blood group system?

☐ homozygous amorph

modifier gene

☐ modifier gene

Match the following causes of the Rh_{null} phenotype:

1   A

2   B

1 ____ ---/---   A   homozygous amorph

2 ____ $X^{o}r$ B   modifier gene

Match the following for the Kell blood group system:

1   B

2   A

1 ____ X^{k} A   amorph

2 ____ K^{o} B   regulator gene

In the Duffy system the amorphic gene is labeled:

☐ *Fy*

☐ *Fy⁰*

☐ *Fyˣ*

A minus-minus phenotype in the Kidd system appears to be caused by a:

☐ homozygous amorph.

☐ modifier gene.

Match the following for the Lutheran system:

1 _____ *In(Lu)*   A   amorph

2 _____ *Lu*   B   modifier gene

Multiple, paired allelic genes which are closely linked are called a gene

complex or gene _____ .

When a modifier gene suppresses the expression of a blood group, it suppresses

☐ only one

☐ all

of the genes in a gene cluster.

When the amorph K^o (or *Lu*) is present as a heterozygote

☐ only one gene cluster

☐ the gene clusters of both chromosomes

fail(s) to make antigen.

The Xgᵃ antigen is known to be controlled by a gene on the _____ chromosome.

Chapter Three:
The ABO System

Objectives for Chapter Three

Upon completion of this chapter you should be able to:

3.1   • **Explain the importance of ABO grouping**

3.2   • **Explain the difference between red cell grouping and reverse grouping**

       • **List the results of both red cell grouping and reverse grouping for each of the ABO blood groups**

       • **Describe the purpose of reagent controls and procedural controls in blood grouping**

3.3   • **Explain how each of the following can cause problems in ABO grouping:**
- inheritance of a rare gene
- mixed populations of cells
- decreased transferase levels
- alteration of blood group antigens by bacterial enzymes
- polyagglutination of red cells
- decreased production of IgM
- unexpected alloagglutinins

3.1

What is the importance of ABO grouping?

ABO grouping is the most important laboratory test performed on potential transfusion recipients and blood donors. The critical nature of ABO grouping stems from two characteristics of the system. First, unlike other blood group systems, antibodies of the ABO system are present in the serum of almost every person who does not have the corresponding antigen. Second, the **alloagglutinins** of the ABO system fix complement and are capable of causing intravascular hemolysis of incompatible red cells. For these reasons, an error in ABO grouping of a patient or donor could be fatal in a transfusion setting. While the crossmatch affords an additional measure of protection, this may not be done in every case.

3.1 QUESTIONS

Which blood group is most important in blood transfusion?

ABO

☐ ABO

☐ Rh

List two reasons why ABO grouping is so important:

Anti-A and/or anti-B are present in the serum of almost every person.

1 _____

_____

_____

ABO antibodies fix complement and can cause intravascular hemolysis.

2 _____

_____

_____

An error in ABO grouping

can

☐ can

☐ cannot

be fatal in a transfusion setting.

The crossmatch affords an additional measure of

protection

_____ .

3.2

What tests are used to determine a person's ABO group?

Accurate determination of a person's ABO group requires two different test procedures: **red cell grouping** (sometimes called **forward grouping**) and **reverse grouping** (sometimes called **serum grouping**). The individual is first assigned to one of four ABO blood groups — A, B, AB or O — based on the reaction of his or her red cells with Blood Grouping Sera Anti-A and Anti-B. Blood Grouping Sera Anti-A and Anti-B are prepared from the sera of group B persons and group A persons, respectively. Anti-A,B serum — prepared from specially selected group O individuals — is not a simple mixture of anti-A and anti-B but is the component of group O serum that has the special property of reacting with weak antigens on the red cells, especially weak A antigens. For this reason Blood Grouping Serum Anti-A,B is used routinely in some laboratories. In others, it is used only for special testing. Anti-A,B serum will agglutinate group A, group B and group AB cells, but not cells of group O. This reagent is especially important when testing donor units to prevent mistyping a weak subgroup and labeling the unit group O. Anti-A,B serum should always be included in resolving discrepant results between cell and serum grouping.

Assuming the tests are properly performed, visible interaction with antiserum (agglutination of the cells) indicates that the cells possess the antigen against which the antiserum is directed. Conversely, no visible interaction indicates that the cells lack the antigen. Table 3.2A shows the results of tests of the red cells of each of the four ABO groups with anti-A and anti-B. About 41 percent of the United States population possess only A antigen, 9 percent have only B antigen, 4 percent have both A and B antigens, while the remaining 46 percent have neither A nor B antigens.

Table 3.2A Incidence of ABO blood groups in the United States.

Red Cells Tested With:		Blood Group	% Incidence
Anti-A	**Anti-B**		
+	Neg.	A	41
Neg.	+	B	9
+	+	AB	4
Neg.	Neg.	O	46

Following or simultaneously with red cell grouping, the serum of the individual is tested with known group A and group B red cells to demonstrate the presence or absence of anti-A and/or anti-B. Because of the similarity in structure between A and B antigens of red cells and antigens of bacteria and plants, virtually everyone who lacks either one or both of the antigens A and B produces antibody to the foreign antigen(s). Antibodies produced as a result of exposure to antigens of bacteria and plants are not observed until four to six months of age. The anti-A and anti-B found in the serum of newborns is of maternal origin. The expected regularly-occurring anti-A and/or anti-B, found in the serum of all people except those of group AB, afford an ideal check on the red cell group. It is desirable to use A_1 cells for maximum reactivity of the regularly-occurring anti-A in group B and group O sera. Some workers use A_2 in addition to A_1 cells. Table 3.2B shows the results expected in red cell grouping and reverse grouping for the four ABO blood groups. Note the reciprocal relationship of the antigens and antibodies, characteristic of the ABO system. Any discrepancy between the results of red cell grouping and reverse grouping must be investigated and resolved before conclusions are drawn as to the individual's true ABO group.

Table 3.2B Results of red cell grouping and reverse grouping for the ABO blood groups.

Cells of Person Tested With:		Red Cell Group	Serum of Person Tested With:		Reverse Group
Anti-A	Anti-B		A_1 Cells	B Cells	
+	Neg.	A	Neg.	+	A
Neg.	+	B	+	Neg.	B
+	+	AB	Neg.	Neg.	AB
Neg.	Neg.	O	+	+	O

In ABO grouping, the antisera used contain IgM antibodies in a low-protein diluent. As described in Focus Question 1.6, the structure of IgM is such that it can cross-link red cells suspended in saline. Agglutination of saline-suspended red cells by IgM anti-A and/or anti-B occurs at room temperature and is virtually immediate. The rapid reaction, requiring no incubation, is due not only to the nature and amount of the antibody in the antiserum, but also to the fact that A and B antigens are present on the red cells in very large numbers. For ABO red cell grouping, the properties of antigen and antibody allow the use of either slide or tube techniques. However, reverse grouping must be done by the more sensitive test tube method because the level of antibody in the serum of any one individual may be low.

Additional Tests Required under Special Circumstances

More extensive testing is required whenever there is disagreement between the red cell group and the reverse group, or when the red cells react weakly with an antiserum. Additional reagents can be used, test conditions can be modified in terms of temperature, and tests of saliva may be helpful. The objective of additional testing is to determine whether one is dealing with a technical problem or an abnormal blood sample from a patient or donor. The results of controls, both reagent and procedural, help in defining the cause of an unusual test result.

Controls in ABO Grouping

Reagent controls for ABO grouping need not be set up separately; they can be an integral part of the test system. The purpose of doing both cell grouping and reverse grouping is for each to confirm the results of the other. If the red cell and reverse group do not correspond, the discrepancy may be related to the reagents used; however, reagents are rarely the source of the problem, especially if other samples being tested do not show discrepant results. When many blood samples are tested simultaneously, problems with reagent sera or reagent red cells will be immediately evident in the form of numerous discrepant results. When only a few blood samples are being tested, one may wish to set up separate controls at the beginning of each day. These controls could consist of known group A and group B cells tested with Blood Grouping Sera Anti-A and Anti-B. This cross-testing confirms the suitability of both reagent red cells and the reagent antisera.

Procedural controls show whether the method and conditions selected (such as temperature and centrifugation) were appropriate for the test system. Provided that cell grouping and reverse grouping match, there is no need to set up separate procedural controls. If no reactions are observed with group O cells, any reaction observed with A or B cells used in reverse grouping is most likely due to anti-A or anti-B. Conversely, if there are reactions with group O cells, any unexpected reactions with A or B cells are probably due to the same cause and must be further investigated.

3.2 QUESTIONS

Name the two tests required to determine an individual's ABO group:

1 _____

2 _____

List the four ABO blood groups:

1 _____

2 _____

3 _____

4 _____

Match the following:

1 _____ Blood Grouping   A   prepared from
         Serum Anti-A   group A persons

2 _____ Blood Grouping   B   prepared from
         Serum Anti-B   group B persons

3 _____ Blood Grouping   C   prepared from
         Serum Anti-A,B   group O persons

List the ABO group of cells that will be agglutinated by Blood Grouping Serum Anti-A,B:

_____

_____

Match the following results of a blood grouping test with the appropriate conclusion:

1 _____ agglutination   A   the cells do not possess the
                                      antigen against which the
                                      antiserum is directed

2 _____ no visible   B   the cells do possess the
         interaction   antigen against which the
                                      antiserum is directed

For each of the following red cell groups, list the ABO antibodies which would be expected in the serum of an adult:

group A _____

group B _____

group AB _____

group O _____

Match the following:

1 ____ forward grouping

A detecting anti-A and/or anti-B in the patient's serum using reagent red cells

2 ____ reverse grouping

B detecting red cell antigens using antisera containing anti-A and anti-B

The origin of ABO antibodies present in a one-month-old infant is the

☐ infant's

☐ mother's

immune system.

Blood Grouping Sera Anti-A and Anti-B used in ABO grouping contain:

☐ IgG antibodies.

☐ IgM antibodies.

The A and B antigens are present in very

☐ small

☐ large

numbers on red cells.

fast, requiring no incubation.

In ABO grouping, the reaction is:

☐ slow, requiring an incubation period of one hour.

☐ fast, requiring no incubation.

When a discrepancy arises between a patient's red cell group and the reverse group:

☐ the patient's red cell group rather than the reverse group is used to match the patient with an appropriate donor.

additional tests must be performed to clarify the discrepancy.

☐ additional tests must be performed to clarify the discrepancy.

In ABO grouping, reagent controls can be part of

the test system

_____

separately

or may be set up _____.

Controls on the method and conditions used in a test system are called:

☐ systematic controls.

procedural controls.

☐ procedural controls.

3.3

What are the potential problems in ABO grouping?

Weak or **mixed-field agglutination** in ABO grouping or disagreement between the red cell group and reverse group may indicate a genetic variant or a change due to disease. More importantly, recent transfusion or fetal-maternal hemorrhage may explain these observations. It is essential that any unusual findings be reported and their cause(s) be identified; otherwise transfusion therapy may be withheld unnecessarily or an incorrect blood group selected for the patient.

A discrepancy between red cell grouping and reverse grouping or an unusual result in red cell testing is probably not due to a technical problem. It may be explained by one or more of the following situations:

- The sample is from an individual who inherited a rare gene (or genes).

- The blood contains more than one population of red cells.

- Transferase levels may be abnormal in association with disease or pregnancy.

- Blood group antigens may be altered by bacterial enzymes.

- Production of IgM may be impaired.

- IgM of specificity other than anti-A and anti-B may be interfering with the test.

By looking at the total picture, i.e., cell and serum test results and the history of the patient or donor, one may obtain clues to the reason for unusual ABO test results. Tests to differentiate and resolve ABO problems and the selection of appropriate blood for transfusion are described in other publications, some of which are included in the Sources of Additional Information at the end of this book.

Weak Antigen Test Results Due to Inheritance

Strong reactions are expected when testing red cells of groups A, B and AB with reagent antisera. Weak agglutination in red cell grouping may indicate that the blood is from an individual who belongs to a subgroup of A or B. This is the most likely explanation when weak reactions are noted in a healthy person such as a blood donor. As mentioned previously, Blood Grouping Serum Anti-A,B will detect some subgroups of A and B which do not react with anti-A or anti-B reagents. In donors, the danger is that subgroups of A (or subgroups of B, though these are very rare) may be mistyped and the unit labeled group O.

Subgroups of A are more of a problem than subgroups of B because they are more common and because of the possible presence of anti-A_1 in the serum of A_2 or A_2B persons. Among Caucasians about 80 percent of those inheriting an A gene produce a straightforward, clearly demonstrable A antigen called A_1. About 20 percent show varying degrees of expression of the A gene. These variations in antigen strength can result from a different form of the transferase, an altered substrate (i.e., H chain) or an absence of the H chain. Most non-A_1 red cells fall into the category of A_2 and are easily identified. The A_2 gene-specified transferase is quantitatively and qualitatively different from the A_1 transferase. There is about one-fifth the quantity of the A_2 transferase in A_2 individuals when compared to A_1 transferase in A_1 individuals. In laboratory experiments, A_1 transferases and A_2 transferases have different requirements of pH and cations for optimum activity. Both transfer N-acetylgalactosamine to the H chain but the A_2 transferase does so less efficiently. For this reason not all the H chains on the red blood cells are converted to A chains. This explains why anti-H sera react more strongly with A_2 red cells than with A_1 cells but less strongly than with O cells. On group O cells, all chains remain as H chains; on group A_1 cells, most chains have a terminal N-acetylgalactosamine, leaving few, if any, unconverted H chains. On A_2 cells, only some of the H chains are altered by the addition of an A sugar, leaving the rest to react with anti-H.

Because persons with A_2 and A_2B cells have a weak A antigen, they sometimes produce an antibody of anti-A specificity which reacts only with the strong A antigen of A_1 or A_1B cells. This is called anti-A_1. It is not entirely clear at this time whether anti-A_1 is a distinct specificity or simply an antibody that "fits" poorly; i.e., it has a low affinity for its antigen and therefore reacts with A_1 cells because they are more densely populated with A antigen than are A_2 cells.

Lectins are seed extracts that agglutinate human red blood cells with a high degree of specificity. Anti-A_1 **lectin** is prepared from the seeds of *Dolichos biflorus*. The reagent can be prepared so that it agglutinates A_1 and A_1B cells but does not agglutinate A_2 or A_2B cells or those of the weaker subgroups of A and AB. Cells which are agglutinated by anti-A_1 lectin but which react weakly or not at all with human anti-A_1 serum are classified as A intermediates.

Subgroups of A weaker than A_2 are rare and they are mainly of academic interest when found in patients. If a patient who is a weak subgroup of A is mistyped as O and given O blood, no serious consequences would be expected. On the other hand weakened A antigens of a donor could cause problems if the blood is mistyped and given to a group O patient. Red cells of the subgroup A_3 are discussed in the section on mixed-field agglutination. Other subgroups result from a variety of gene interactions and will not be discussed here.

Another inherited trait which interferes with red cell grouping is Cad. Cad positive cells are polyagglutinable. A more detailed discussion of this very rare phenomenon is included later in this focus question.

Mixed Populations of Cells

Mixed-field agglutination in ABO grouping usually indicates transfusion with blood of a different group, such as group O to group A, or more significantly, group A to group O. Because of the serious nature of blood transfusions of ABO group other than the patient's own, it is extremely important to resolve the cause of mixed-field agglutination prior to transfusion. To assume that a patient is group A or B because some of the cells in his or her circulation are A or B could lead to disastrous consequences. An investigation of the patient's history may help to verify the cause of the mixed-field agglutination. If recent transfusions and fetal-maternal hemorrhage can be conclusively ruled out, other causes should be considered — **chimera**, subgroup A$_3$, **leukemia** and Tn **polyagglutination**.

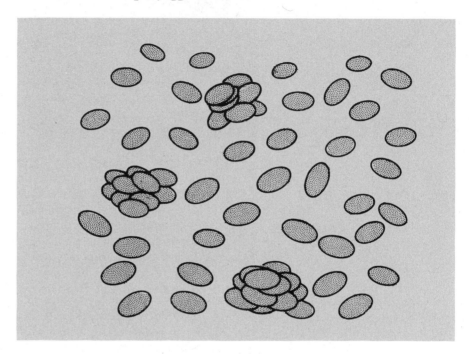

Figure 3.3A Mixed-field agglutination. Small, tightly agglutinated cells in a field of unagglutinated cells. The number of cells in each clump and the number of clumps will depend on the cause of the mixed-field agglutination.

Blood group chimeras most often result from exchange of primordial blood cells during early fetal life of non-identical twins. As a result of this exchange, two distinct types of red blood cells (and leukocytes) may be observed. History of twinning in the family is suggestive evidence that the patient may be a blood group chimera. If both twins are available for testing, the proportion of the two red cell populations observed in one twin may bear no relation to the proportion observed in the other. Further evidence of chimerism is obtained if tests for other blood groups also show mixed-field agglutination in the same proportion of positive to negative as was observed in ABO testing. Test results of parents and children of the person may determine which blood group is from the person's own **genome** and which has been derived from the twin.

The subgroup A$_3$ characteristically shows a mixed-field agglutination with Blood Grouping Serum Anti-A. However, all A$_3$ cells, even those not agglutinated by anti-A, carry some A antigen. Although A$_3$

is an inherited trait, the transferases that produce it are not always the same. Some persons whose red cells are A_3 have an A_1 transferase and others have a transferase with A_2 characteristics. Anti-A_1 is rarely found in the serum of a person with A_3 red cells.

While polyagglutinable cells due to Tn activation often show mixed-field agglutination, it seems more appropriate to discuss Tn-activated cells with the other types of polyagglutination. Very strong reactions with anti-A_1 lectin (*Dolichos biflorus*) and the presence of a normal anti-A in the serum lead to the suspicion that the cells are Tn-activated.

Decreased Transferase Levels

Occasionally, a sample from a patient with acute leukemia may appear to contain red cell populations of two different blood groups because some cells have lost all the original antigen while others retain small amounts. During the course of the disease, reactivity of the cells may become progressively weaker and, in extreme cases, cells from group A or group B patients appear to be group O. This has been shown to result from lowered transferase levels. When the patient is in remission, the red cell type may revert to normal. When red cells show unusually weak or mixed-field agglutination with anti-A or anti-B, or an apparent group O patient reverse groups as A or B, information as to the clinical diagnosis should be sought. If acute leukemia is the diagnosis, additional testing will be necessary to determine the patient's true group prior to transfusion. This could be either a group A patient whose A antigen has diminished or a group O patient who is producing too little anti-A to be detectable. The latter is not likely unless the anti-B is also weakened or missing. In patients with leukemia not only are transferase levels sometimes lower than normal but immunoglobulin levels are also frequently reduced; both anti-A and anti-B are affected.

Transferase levels are weakened during pregnancy and this can result in weaker reactions with anti-A and anti-B when testing the red cells of obstetrical patients. In actual practice this is rarely observed, but an excess of apparently A_2 individuals among obstetrical patients has been reported.

Blood Group Antigens Altered by Bacterial Enzymes

Some group A individuals with intestinal obstruction, carcinoma of the colon or rectum, and other disorders of the lower intestine acquire a B-like antigen. The reaction observed between anti-B and the acquired B antigen is usually weak and often disperses easily. Increased permeability of the intestinal wall allows the passage of bacterial enzymes into the circulation. These enzymes act on the terminal sugar of the A antigen, causing the patient's red cells to be agglutinated by anti-B (in addition to their original reactivity with anti-A, which is unaffected). The A sugar, N-acetylgalactosamine, is deacetylated by the enzyme to form D-galactosamine which is very similar to D-galactose, the B sugar. However, on reverse grouping, the results observed are those expected of a group A person; that is, only anti-B is present in the serum. If the intestinal condition improves, the red cells revert to normal and no longer react with anti-B.

Whereas polyagglutination of red blood cells has no direct relationship to the ABO system, it is discussed here because it is most often initially observed when testing with anti-A and anti-B. Many forms of polyagglutination have been described but those that are most thoroughly understood are T, Tn, Tk and Cad. Each of these forms can cause discrepant reactions when testing with anti-A and/or anti-B reagents. T and Tk polyagglutinability result from the exposure of T and Tk red cell receptors. Each receptor (antigen) can then react with its respective antibody (anti-T and anti-Tk) normally present in sera from most adults. The T or Tk receptors on the cells are exposed by the action of bacterial enzymes either *in vivo* or sometimes *in vitro*. Interference in ABO testing arises because commercially prepared anti-A and anti-B are not highly diluted and thus may contain weak anti-T and anti-Tk. In addition, anti-T and anti-Tk are IgM cold **agglutinins** reacting best by the same methods used for ABO testing. The reactions observed are usually weak but at times may be as strong as the expected reaction of an A cell with anti-A. Polyagglutination should be suspected if both an antigen and the corresponding antibody appear to be present in the same blood sample. It is common for cells with an "acquired B" antigen to be T-activated also. Apparently the same organism produces both enzymes which cause these phenomena.

The least understood of the polyagglutinable cells are Tn-activated cells. The cause or causes for the activation of Tn on red cells is not clear. Not only are the red blood cells affected, but most patients also have a neutropenia and thrombocytopenia. It has been suggested that the cells are affected in the bone marrow, some being Tn-activated and others not. Mixed-field agglutination may be seen in tests with anti-A and anti-B, but this is due to anti-Tn found in the sera of donors used to prepare anti-A and anti-B sera. In addition, certain lectins, such as *Dolichos biflorus*, have a specific affinity for the Tn receptor; consequently, Tn-activated cells always appear to be strongly A_1 positive when tested with this lectin. This affinity of Tn for *Dolichos biflorus* has led to the designation "acquired A." See Table 3.3B for the reactions of other lectins with polyagglutinable cells.

Table 3.3B Forms of polyagglutination and the expected reactions with some lectins.

Lectins	T	Tk	Tn	Cad
Arachis hypogaea	+	+	o	o
Salvia sclarea	o	o	+	o
Salvia horminum	o	o	+	+
Dolichos biflorus	o*	o*	+	+
Glycine soja	+	o	+	+

*Not true for A_1 cells because *Dolichos biflorus* is anti-A_1.

Cad positive red blood cells are very rare. The Cad positive trait is inherited and the antibody that reacts with Cad positive red blood cells is found in most adult sera. This antibody has the same specificity as anti-Sd^a, but the relationship of Cad and Sd^a antigens is not clear. It has been suggested that Cad is a "super Sd(a+)," but not all evidence supports this. The agglutination which results from reacting anti-Sd^a with random cells will range from weak to strong and may have a mixed-field appearance.

IgM Levels

As described earlier, the alloagglutinins of the ABO system are predominantly IgM. If anti-A and/or anti-B are expected in a person's serum and cannot be demonstrated, it may indicate lower than normal production of IgM by the patient or donor. IgM levels are very low at birth; however, the newborn can produce limited quantities of IgM. Levels of IgM increase gradually during the first 18 months of life and generally decrease in old age. The titer of ABO alloagglutinins reflects these changes. The body's ability to produce IgM can also be affected by disease and by immunosuppressive drugs. Thus, when expected alloagglutinins are weak or absent, information as to the age and diagnosis of the individual being tested is required. If the sample is from a newborn infant or an elderly person, failure to reverse group as expected is probably simply a reflection of age. A diagnosis of **hypogammaglobulinemia** or leukemia is consistent with decreased immunoglobulin production. When testing babies, elderly persons, or patients with diseases in which IgM levels are known to be lower than normal, the reverse group may be misleading. Under these circumstances, the only alternative is to rely on the results of red cell tests.

Occasionally, the expected alloagglutinins are not demonstrable in the sera or plasma of healthy adults. While this may have no significance, it could indicate that the corresponding antigen is present on the person's red cells. A weak reaction in red cell testing may have been overlooked because test tubes were shaken too vigorously or slide tests were read too hastily. Alternatively, the antigen may be so weak that it requires special reagents or techniques to be detected.

Unexpected Alloagglutinins

If a serum or plasma reacts with A$_1$ and B cells but the red cells do not appear to be group O, it is highly probable that the reaction is due to an unexpected alloantibody rather than due to anti-A or anti-B. Any antibody which can agglutinate saline-suspended cells at room temperature could react with reverse grouping cells if they carry the appropriate antigen. Anti-M, anti-P$_1$, anti-A$_1$ and anti-Lewis interfere with reverse grouping occasionally; but from an economic standpoint it is not feasible for manufacturers to select A and B cells that are exclusively M negative, P$_1$ negative and Lewis negative. If a serum reacts with group O screening cells when tested under the same conditions as A or B cells, it contains an unexpected antibody which may account for the agglutination of the reverse grouping cells. If screening cells are not agglutinated by the serum, any reactivity with A or B cells is almost certainly due to anti-A or anti-B. If the cells are group A, the most likely explanation is anti-A$_1$ in the serum of a subgroup of A. A less likely possibility is an antibody directed against an antigen that has a low incidence in the general population but is, by chance, present on the A or B cells. The presence of anti-A$_1$ should be confirmed by testing with additional A$_1$, A$_2$ and O cells as described in other publications.

3.3 QUESTIONS

When testing group A, B or AB red cells with Blood Grouping Sera Anti-A and Anti-B,

☐ weak

☐ strong

reactions are expected.

Weak reactions in red cell grouping a healthy person may indicate:

☐ a subgroup of A or B.

☐ high ABO antigen density.

When testing the cells of donors, the danger is that subgroups of A or B may be mistyped and labeled group _____ .

Which are more common?

☐ subgroups of A

☐ subgroups of B

The majority of Caucasians inheriting an A gene produce a normal A antigen called:

☐ A_1

☐ A_2

True or false:

The A_1 transferase is produced in a greater amount than the A_2 transferase.

_____

The A_1 transferase is more efficient than the A_2 transferase.

_____

The two transferases require the same pH and cations for optimal *in vitro* activity.

_____

Match the following:

1 ____ group A$_1$ cells   A   react strongly
with anti-H sera

2 ____ group A$_2$ cells   B   react intermediately
with anti-H sera

3 ____ group O cells   C   react weakly with
anti-H sera

People with A$_2$ or A$_2$B cells may produce:

☐ anti-A$_1$.

☐ anti-A$_2$.

Extracts of seeds which agglutinate human red cells with a high degree

of specificity are called _____ .

Red cells which react weakly or not at all with human anti-A$_1$ serum
but which are agglutinated by anti-A$_1$ lectin are called

_____ .

Patients who have been transfused with blood of an ABO group

other than their own ABO group may show _____
agglutination.

Chimeras most often arise from:

☐ fetal-maternal exchange of blood cells.

☐ exchange of primordial blood cells between non-identical twins
early in fetal life.

Mixed-field agglutination is

☐ characteristically

☐ rarely

seen when testing subgroup A$_3$ with anti-A.

weaker	In leukemia, A and/or B antigens may become progressively
	☐ stronger
	☐ weaker
	but revert to normal during remission.
	Bacterial enzymes may cause group A people to acquire:
	☐ new B antigens.
altered antigens very similar to B antigens.	☐ altered antigens very similar to B antigens.
	T or Tk receptors on red cells may be exposed by:
	☐ complement fixation.
bacterial enzymes.	☐ bacterial enzymes.
	Anti-T and anti-Tk are:
	☐ IgG antibodies.
IgM antibodies.	☐ IgM antibodies.
	The Cad positive trait is:
inherited.	☐ inherited.
	☐ acquired.
	The antibody which reacts with Cad positive cells has the same
anti-Sd^a	specificity as _____ .
	The mixed-field agglutination seen when testing Tn-activated red cells with anti-A and anti-B is due to their reaction with:
	☐ anti-A or anti-B.
anti-Tn.	☐ anti-Tn.

decrease.
are
unexpected alloantibodies.

In leukemia or hypogammaglobulinemia, the patient's ABO antibody levels would be expected to:

☐ increase.

☐ decrease.

Levels of anti-A and anti-B

☐ are

☐ are not

expected to vary depending upon the patient's age.

When a patient's serum reacts with A_1 and B cells but his or her red cells do not appear to be group O, the reaction is most likely due to:

☐ the presence of anti-A and anti-B antibodies.

☐ unexpected alloantibodies.

Chapter Four:
The Rh System and Rh Typing

Objectives for Chapter Four

Upon completion of this chapter you should be able to:

4.1
- Explain the importance of Rh typing

- Describe the two most common ways for an Rh negative individual to be exposed to Rh positive red cells

- Describe how Rh immunization can be suppressed

4.2
- Describe the difference between the two major kinds of Rh antisera, as defined by the nature of their diluents

- Describe Blood Grouping Serum Anti-D (Anti-Rh_o) for Saline Tube Test

- Explain how IgG antibodies can be chemically modified to agglutinate red cells suspended in saline

- Describe Blood Grouping Serum Anti-D (Anti-Rh_o) for Slide and Modified Tube Tests

- Describe Blood Grouping Serum Anti-D (Anti-Rh_o) MAGNASERA for Slide and Rapid Tube Tests

4.3
- List the circumstances in which D^u testing is done and explain its importance

- Explain how an Rh phenotype is established

4.4
- List the two categories of problems in Rh typing

- Explain the causes of unusually weak agglutination and positive controls in Rh typing

4.1

What is the importance of Rh typing?

The Rh-hr system includes many antigens but the major one is D, alternatively referred to as Rh_o. The term Rh positive is used to denote red cells that carry the D (Rh_o) antigen or its variant D^u. Red cells that have neither D nor D^u on their membranes are termed Rh negative. With the exception of A and B, the most important of all blood group antigens is undoubtedly D. This is because the consequences of the presence of anti-D can be tragic: transfusion reactions due to Rh antibodies can be severe and Rh hemolytic disease of the newborn can be a heartbreaking experience. However, unlike the situation in the ABO system, an Rh negative person does not usually have anti-D in his or her serum. Rh antigens are confined to red cells and are not found in body fluids or natural substances; therefore, exposure to red cells is the only way a person can become immunized to Rh. Also contributing to the importance of the Rh system is the fact that the D antigen is one of the most effective blood group immunogens. Because of the clinical implications, a discussion of Rh antibodies and how they are stimulated will precede information concerning testing for Rh antigens.

As stated above, no natural substances chemically similar to the D antigen have been found; therefore when an Rh negative person is found to have anti-D, that individual has invariably been exposed to Rh positive red cells. The two most likely ways for Rh positive red cells to reach the circulation of an Rh negative individual are:

- Transfusion of red cells from an Rh positive donor to an Rh negative recipient. Except in rare circumstances, this is contrary to good transfusion practice; therefore it is usually the result of clerical or technical error.

- Passage of red cells from an Rh positive fetus through the placenta to the Rh negative mother. This almost always occurs to some extent at delivery and occasionally late in pregnancy.

The number of persons immunized to D as a result of fetal-maternal passage of red cells has decreased rapidly in recent years. Although we know of no way to prevent fetal red cells from reaching the mother, her response to the antigen can be suppressed with proper treatment. Rh immune globulin has been available for postpartum administration since 1968 but, regrettably, it is still not used in every situation where it is needed. Many circumstances can lead to Rh immunization, such as early abortions, traumatic accidents during pregnancy, and **amniocentesis**. Also, a small number of women are immunized by fetal red cells which traverse the placenta during the last trimester of pregnancy. Rh immune globulin may now be given antepartum and, unless this is done, 1 to 2 percent of Rh negative women will continue to be immunized despite proper postpartum treatment.

The formation of anti-D as a result of accidental transfusion of Rh positive red cells to an Rh negative recipient is also decreasing. This is due to increased attention to the performance of testing procedures and techniques but, here again, there is still room for improvement. Accidental transfusion of Rh positive blood to an Rh negative person need not result in antibody production if the accident is discovered in time, since immunization can be prevented by the administration of an adequate dose of Rh immune globulin.

Blood component therapy is another potential source of immunization to red cell antigens. Platelet or **granulocyte** preparations are not entirely free of intact red cells or **stroma**. Because it is often not practical to match the Rh antigens of platelet donors with those of the patient, some authorities advocate the administration of Rh immune globulin when platelets from Rh positive donors are infused into Rh negative patients. Granulocyte transfusions should be both ABO and Rh compatible due to the large number of red cells introduced with the granulocytes. A more complete discussion of the immune response and its prevention is found in Chapter Eight.

The entire burden of preventing the formation of anti-D as a result of transfusion lies in accurate testing of the red cells of both patient and donor. If anti-D is already present in the serum of an Rh negative patient, it is even more critical that Rh typing of potential donors be correct since administration of Rh positive blood to a patient whose serum contains anti-D may cause a severe or even fatal transfusion reaction. For these reasons, it is recommended that Rh tests on patients be done in duplicate using two different kinds of reagents.

4.1 QUESTIONS

The major antigen of the Rh-hr system is the D antigen, which is also

called the _____ antigen.

Match the following:

1 ____ Rh positive   A   D antigen or D^u present on red cell membranes

2 ____ Rh negative   B   neither D antigen nor D^u is present on red cell membranes

An Rh negative person would normally

☐ be expected

☐ not be expected

to have anti-D in his serum.

The D antigen is a:

☐ weak immunogen.

☐ strong immunogen.

Natural substances chemically similar to the D antigen

☐ have

☐ have not

been found.

What are the two ways in which an Rh negative person can be exposed to D antigen?

1 _____

_____

2 _____

_____

Margin answers (left column):

Rh_o

1 A

2 B

not be expected

strong immunogen.

have not

transfusion with Rh positive blood

passage of Rh positive fetal cells to an Rh negative mother

Rh negative patients

☐ are

are not ☐ are not

commonly transfused with Rh positive blood.

Fetal-maternal passage of red cells usually occurs:

☐ in the first trimester.

in the third trimester and ☐ in the third trimester and especially at delivery.
especially at delivery.

In recent years, the number of women immunized to D by fetal-maternal passage of red cells has substantially:

decreased. ☐ decreased.

☐ increased.

Immunization by Rh positive cells at delivery is suppressed by:

☐ preventing the passage of red cells from the fetal to the maternal circulation.

postpartum administration ☐ postpartum administration of Rh immune globulin.
of Rh immune globulin.

Rh immunization due to fetal-maternal passage of cells as a result of trauma during pregnancy can be suppressed by

antepartum administration _____ .
of Rh immune globulin

Rh immunization due to fetal-maternal hemorrhage in the last trimester

antepartum administration of pregnancy can be prevented by _____
of Rh immune globulin

_____ .

If an Rh negative person is accidentally transfused with Rh positive

administration of an blood, immunization can be suppressed by _____
adequate dose of Rh
immune globulin _____ .

Granulocyte transfusions should be both ABO and Rh compatible because:

☐ granulocytes carry Rh antigens.

☐ large numbers of red cells are introduced with the granulocytes.

Platelet preparations

☐ are

☐ are not

entirely free of red cells.

In an Rh negative person who has already been Rh immunized, transfusion with Rh positive cells may lead to _____ .

large numbers of red cells are introduced with the granulocytes.

are not

a severe or fatal transfusion reaction

4.2

What are the tests and reagents used to determine an individual's Rh type?

The presence or absence of the D (Rh$_o$) antigen is demonstrated by testing the red cells with Blood Grouping Serum Anti-D (Anti-Rh$_o$). A positive reaction, i.e., agglutination of the cells by the antibody, indicates that the cells have D antigen; if the cells are not agglutinated by anti-D, they lack D antigen. Red cells that are not agglutinated by anti-D in initial testing may be further tested for D^u. For reasons discussed later, this test is always done on donor blood; the policy on testing patients for D^u varies from one institution to another. Tests for other antigens of the Rh system (C, c, E and e) are performed less frequently, but the principle of the procedure is the same as for D. The actual procedure and how it is controlled depend on the kind of Rh antiserum that is selected.

Rh typing reagents can be divided into two general groups according to the nature of their diluents. Antisera prepared in low-protein diluents without potentiators are the least likely to cause false positive agglutination. Because low-protein reagents can be used with washed red cells suspended in saline, problems created by abnormalities of the patient's serum can be avoided. Cells with a positive direct antiglobulin test can also be tested more accurately with low-protein reagents. False positive agglutination is most often due to cross-linking of red blood cells that have been sensitized (usually *in vivo*) prior to the addition of the antiserum. High concentrations of protein and synthetic potentiators, such as **polyvinylpyrrolidone (PVP)**, exacerbate cross-linking. To facilitate recognition of false positive results in Rh typing — especially when testing patients — controls are required. With low-protein antisera (6 to 8 percent protein) ABO grouping performed concomitantly with Rh typing can serve as the control. With high-protein antisera (above 10 percent protein) a parallel control must be set up with every test. The parallel control consists of the same cell suspension, tested with the diluent used by the manufacturer in preparing the Rh antiserum.

It is extremely important *always to follow the manufacturer's directions* enclosed with each reagent. Each time a new lot number of antiserum is to be used, it is essential to check for the appropriate control, the number of drops of cells and of reagent, the necessary red blood cell suspending medium, and whether or not incubation is required. Be aware that manufacturers change directions from time to time. If these changes reflect changes in the reagent, the test results may be affected if the reagent is used according to the previous directions.

The following paragraphs describe commercially prepared Rh antisera. The different antisera contain antibodies with the same specificity but different reactivity. The selection of one over others is a matter of personal preference, availability and test technique.

Blood Grouping Serum Anti-D (Anti-Rh$_o$) for Saline Tube Test

A reagent labeled "For Saline Tube Test" may be used only in a test tube while other Rh antisera can be used in slide test techniques as well as tube techniques. To prepare this reagent, IgM anti-D is used and only minimal quantities of bovine albumin are added to stabilize the antibody; thus this is a low-protein antiserum. IgM saline tube test anti-D agglutinates saline-suspended D positive cells after incubation at 37°C for 15 to 60 minutes.

Reactions with IgM saline tube test reagents are generally not as strong as with slide/rapid tube test reagents, such as those described below. Furthermore, because raw material for IgM saline tube test antiserum is generally of low potency and is scarce, this reagent is more expensive to manufacture than others.

A major disadvantage of Blood Grouping Serum Anti-D (Anti-Rh$_o$) for Saline Tube Test is that it cannot be used in the test for D^u. Saline-agglutinating IgM antibodies do not remain firmly attached to the red cell during the washing involved in this test because they have a lower affinity for their antigens than do IgG antibodies. Testing for D^u may be accomplished with antisera containing IgG anti-D (either chemically modified or unmodified). Prior to 1979, IgM saline tube test antiserum was the only low-protein antiserum available, but this has been replaced in many laboratories by chemically modified Rh antisera.

Chemically Modified Rh Antisera

It is possible to alter IgG molecules by chemical reduction so that they have some of the properties of IgM antibodies *in vitro*, specifically the ability to agglutinate red cells in saline. In unmodified IgG the distance between the two antigen-binding sites of the antibody is about 24 nm, but if the disulfide bonds at the hinge region are broken, the molecule can open further and span a much larger distance, as shown in Figure 4.2A. This offers a great advantage in preparing reagents because it allows the manufacturer to combine the desirable properties of antisera prepared from IgM (i.e., few false positive results) and the desirable properties of IgG antisera (i.e., rapid reactions).

The first commercially available Rh reagent prepared from chemically reduced IgG anti-D was Blood Grouping Serum Anti-D (Anti-Rh$_o$) NOVASERA for Saline Tube and Slide Tests. This reagent can replace Blood Grouping Serum Anti-D for Saline Tube Test and has all the advantages of Blood Grouping Serum Anti-D for Slide and Modified Tube Tests. NOVASERA Anti-D agglutinates saline-suspended cells without the aid of high concentrations of albumin or other potentiators. Cells from patients with autoimmune disease, which have a positive direct antiglobulin test, can be tested as accurately with NOVASERA Anti-D as with saline tube test (IgM) anti-D.

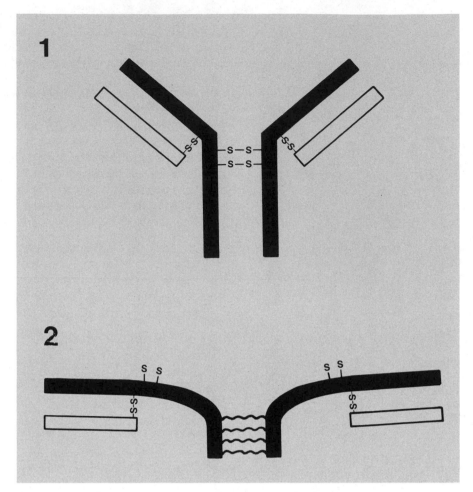

Figure 4.2A (1) An IgG molecule. (2) A chemically reduced IgG molecule. After reducing the disulfide bonds between the heavy chains, other noncovalent bonds (indicated by the wavy lines) continue to hold the heavy chains together. The chemically reduced molecules are subsequently treated to prevent the disulfide bonds from reforming. The distance between antigen-binding sites is now about 400 Å (40 nm).

NOVASERA Anti-D can be used with either serum-suspended or saline-suspended cells. For D (Rh$_o$) typing, incubation at 37°C is not required. For D^u testing, tubes showing no agglutination after centrifugation can be incubated at 37°C and converted to the D^u test, provided the cells have a negative direct antiglobulin test.

No separate control is required if the test using NOVASERA Anti-D is performed and read simultaneously with Blood Grouping Serum Anti-A, Anti-B and/or Anti-A,B. Such concomitant tests can serve as controls for NOVASERA Anti-D and other low-protein Rh antisera because the final composition of the products is serologically similar, containing only minimal protein. Separate controls are unnecessary except when the red cells react with both anti-A and anti-B and the reverse group indicates that the red cell group may be incorrect.

In situations where ABO grouping and Rh typing are not performed by the same technique, any test that will detect spontaneous agglutination of the patient's cells can serve as a control. Such tests include an auto control using the patient's red cells suspended in his or her own serum, or suspended in saline (to duplicate the test situation), or the addition of 6 to 8 percent albumin to the patient's cells.

Blood Grouping Serum Anti-D (Anti-Rh$_o$) for Slide and Modified Tube Tests

In the manufacture of reagents labeled "For Slide and Modified Tube Tests," IgG anti-D, bovine albumin and synthetic potentiators are incorporated into the reagent. These are high-protein reagents which may be used on a slide with whole blood or in a test tube with cells suspended in saline, serum or plasma. Any antiserum prepared in a high-protein diluent may give false positive reactions with serum-suspended cells if the patient's serum is abnormal in some respect. For example, in patients with multiple myeloma and certain other conditions, the normal ratio of serum albumin to serum globulin may be inverted or otherwise abnormal. Cells suspended in abnormal serum, especially when subjected to heat, may aggregate spontaneously (rouleaux) and appear to be agglutinated. To reduce the likelihood of false positive reactions due to serum abnormalities, the patient's cells may be suspended in saline prior to testing. However, even with saline-suspended cells there is the possibility of false positive test results in some patients. Therefore, to confirm the validity of Rh typing using a high-protein reagent, a control is run at the same time as the test. The control reagent, called Rh-hr Control, consists of exactly the same constituents as the anti-D serum, but inert serum is added to the control in place of the anti-D-containing serum used in the reagent (see Figure 4.2B). By performing the control in parallel with the test, agglutination observed in the test and not in the control can be attributed to the antibody component of the anti-D reagent.

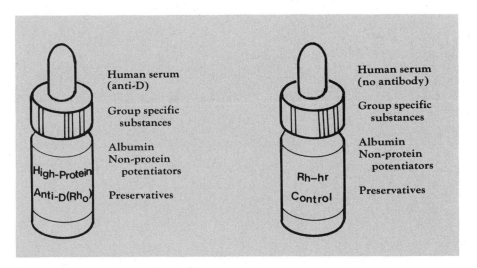

Figure 4.2B When using high-protein anti-D, a parallel control is required. The control should contain the same constituents as the anti-D reagent except for the antibody.

Any reaction caused by the constituents of the suspending medium will be observed in the Rh-hr Control as well as in the test, showing that the test result is invalid. In other words, if the test with anti-D is positive and the Rh-hr Control is negative, the patient is Rh positive; if both tests (anti-D and the Rh-hr Control) are positive, the typing is not reliable. To determine the correct type of the patient, the cells should be washed free of serum and tested with a low-protein antiserum such as Blood Grouping Serum Anti-D (Anti-Rh$_o$) NOVASERA for Saline Tube and Slide Tests or Blood Grouping Serum Anti-D (Anti-Rh$_o$) for Saline Tube Test.

Blood Grouping Serum Anti-D (Anti-Rh$_o$) MAGNASERA for Slide and Rapid Tube Tests and MAGNASERA Control

The advantages of traditional high-protein Rh antisera, such as the reagent just described, are that they provide quick results and, when used in a test tube, the opportunity to perform the D^u test without using additional anti-D. However, because they are extremely viscous, they may cause sticky red cell buttons that are sometimes difficult to resuspend, and negative tests may not have a smooth appearance.

MAGNASERA Anti-D is an improvement over traditional high-protein reagents which contain 25 to 30 percent protein as well as potentiators. MAGNASERA Anti-D is prepared from chemically modified IgG anti-D, which requires dilution in only 15 percent protein. No synthetic potentiators are needed to give rapid, strong reactions. The lowered viscosity of this reagent results in several direct advantages over traditional slide/rapid tube reagents, including faster reactions with slide testing and more compact cell buttons that are easier to resuspend. This is particularly helpful when testing cells with a weaker D antigen because forceful resuspension of the button is not necessary. The advantages of lowered viscosity are most evident when using any of the tube techniques with serum-suspended or plasma-suspended cells.

MAGNASERA Anti-D requires the parallel use of MAGNASERA Control since the protein concentration of the reagent is high enough to cause a false positive result with some Rh negative cells coated with IgG; however, on the basis of protein concentration, fewer false positives would be expected than with traditional high-protein antisera.

4.2 QUESTIONS

The presence or absence of the D antigen is demonstrated by testing

red cells with _____ .

In this test, agglutination indicates a:

☐ positive test.

☐ negative test.

Red cells that are not agglutinated by anti-D may be further tested for what variant of D?

_____

Other antigens of the Rh system

☐ are

☐ are not

routinely tested for.

False positive agglutination of sensitized red cells is more likely to occur with an antiserum prepared in a

☐ low-protein

☐ high-protein

diluent.

In order to recognize false positive test results in Rh typing, it is

important to use _____ .

Blood Grouping Serum Anti-D (Anti-Rh$_o$) for Saline Tube Test is a

☐ low-protein

☐ high-protein

antiserum.

Sidebar answers:

Blood Grouping Serum Anti-D (Anti-Rh$_o$)

positive test.

D^u

are not

high-protein

controls

low-protein

The antibodies in Blood Grouping Serum Anti-D (Anti-Rh_o) for Saline Tube Test are:

☐ IgG antibodies.

☐ IgM antibodies.

IgM antibodies.

Blood Grouping Serum Anti-D (Anti-Rh_o) for Saline Tube Test

☐ can

☐ cannot

cannot

be used to test for D^u.

Chemically modified IgG antibodies in which the disulfide bonds of the hinge region are broken agglutinate red cells without the aid of

high concentrations of albumin or synthetic potentiators

_____

_____ .

Which type of antibody is used in making Blood Grouping Serum Anti-D (Anti-Rh_o) NOVASERA for Saline Tube and Slide Tests?

☐ chemically modified IgG

☐ chemically modified IgM

chemically modified IgG

If tests using NOVASERA Anti-D are performed and read simultaneously with Blood Grouping Sera Anti-A and Anti-B, a separate control:

☐ is required.

☐ is not required.

is not required.

Blood Grouping Serum Anti-D (Anti-Rh_o) for Slide and Modified Tube Tests is a

☐ low-protein

☐ high-protein

high-protein

reagent.

When using an anti-D reagent prepared in a high-protein diluent and serum-suspended cells, a

☐ false positive

☐ false negative

test result may occur if the patient's serum is abnormal.

High-protein anti-D reagents sometimes cause sticky red cell buttons

because of their high ⎯⎯⎯⎯⎯⎯⎯⎯⎯⎯⎯⎯⎯⎯⎯⎯⎯⎯⎯ .

Match the following:

1 ⎯⎯ 15 percent protein   A   traditional high-protein anti-D

2 ⎯⎯ 25 to 30 percent   B   MAGNASERA Anti-D
         protein

Which reagent antiserum has the higher viscosity?

☐ traditional high-protein anti-D

☐ MAGNASERA Anti-D

Which type of antibody is used in making MAGNASERA Anti-D?

☐ chemically modified IgM

☐ chemically modified IgG

4.3

What Rh testing other than D typing is performed and when?

Under some circumstances, blood samples which appear to be D negative are further tested for the variant of the D antigen, D^u. There are also circumstances in which anti-C, -c, -E, and -e reagents may be used.

D^u Testing

Not all red cells can be classified as Rh positive or Rh negative by direct agglutination tests. The cells of a few persons react weakly with anti-D or require a longer reaction time than most Rh positive cells. An even smaller number of persons have red cells that are not agglutinated by anti-D but absorb the antibody. The sensitized cells can then be agglutinated by antiglobulin serum. These cells are called D^u. Cells of the D^u phenotype may fall anywhere within this spectrum of reactivity with anti-D.

Because D^u is a form of D, red cells of the D^u phenotype can stimulate the production of anti-D in Rh negative recipients and, more importantly, react with anti-D *in vivo*. It is for these reasons that donor blood must be shown to be negative not only in the test for D but also in the test for D^u. In general, testing the red cells of recipients for D^u is considered unnecessary. The recipient's welfare is not compromised if he or she is of the D^u phenotype but is typed as D negative and receives Rh negative red cells. In such circumstances Rh negative donor blood may be used unnecessarily.

It is important that the D^u status of the D negative pregnant woman be established early in pregnancy. If the mother is found to be Rh positive, D^u variant, she is not a candidate for Rh immune globulin prophylaxis — either antepartum or postpartum — whereas the Rh negative (D and D^u negative) mother is a candidate. The reason for performing the D^u test early in pregnancy is to avoid misinterpreting the cause of a positive fetal cell screening test at the time of delivery.

In addition to prenatal patients, newborn babies are also tested for D^u if they type as D negative. Again, this relates to the need for Rh immune globulin: the D negative, D^u negative baby cannot immunize its mother; for this reason she does not need Rh immune globulin protection. However, the mother should receive Rh immune globulin if the baby is of the D^u phenotype.

As stated earlier, D^u red cells fall into a wide spectrum of reactivity when tested with anti-D reagents. How each cell is detected depends on the type of anti-D that is used and the kind of test that is performed. To test for D^u, red cells are incubated at 37°C with an IgG anti-D and an antiglobulin test is performed. If serum-suspended cells are used, some blood samples at the upper end of the D^u spectrum will be agglutinated weakly by most anti-D reagents prior to the antiglobulin test, either at room temperature or at 37°C. When the same red cells are suspended in saline, direct agglutination may not be observed, or it may be seen with one reagent and not another. Regardless of whether the red cells are agglutinated directly by anti-D or they absorb anti-D and it is detected in the antiglobulin phase of the test, they are Rh positive, provided both controls (for D typing and the D^u test) are negative. Details of test procedures and proper controls are given in the package inserts that accompany anti-D reagents.

Phenotyping

Establishing the Rh phenotype of an individual allows one to postulate a probable genotype. Information as to the probable genotype is required in parentage testing for medico-legal reasons and in family counseling when the mother is known to have an antibody capable of causing hemolytic disease of the newborn. Results of tests of the father and any previous children may help to predict the likelihood of a child *in utero* (or future children) inheriting the offending gene from the father. The interpretation of test results at the genetic level is discussed following Focus Question 2.8.

Besides their use in establishing a probable genotype, anti-C, -c, -E and -e are also used to test the red cells of patients who have antibodies, either to help identify the antibody or to confirm its apparent specificity. Patients who are likely to receive multiple transfusions in the future may also be typed for C, c, E and e antigens, partly to avoid administration of blood likely to immunize them, but also to establish their phenotypes should they produce an antibody in the future.

4.3 QUESTIONS

Cells which are of the D^u phenotype

☐ can

☐ cannot

stimulate the production of anti-D.

Cells which are not agglutinated by anti-D but absorb the antibody and are detected in the antiglobulin procedure are called

_____ .

It is most important to show that

☐ donor blood

☐ recipient blood

is negative in the tests for both D and D^u.

The D^u status of a pregnant woman who has been typed as D negative should be established

☐ early in pregnancy.

☐ late in pregnancy.

A pregnant woman whose cells are not agglutinated by anti-D but are D^u positive, providing the testing was done early in pregnancy,

☐ is

☐ is not

a candidate for Rh immune globulin.

An Rh negative woman whose baby is of the D^u phenotype

☐ should

☐ should not

receive postpartum Rh immune globulin.

Margin answers:

can

D^u

donor blood

early in pregnancy.

is not

should

On the basis of the Rh phenotype, one

can

☐ can

☐ cannot

postulate the Rh genotype.

The D^u test can be done with:

☐ Blood Grouping Serum Anti-D (Anti-Rh$_o$) for Slide and Modified Tube Tests.

☐ chemically modified anti-D reagents.

both of these reagents   ☐ both of these reagents

4.4

What problems occur in Rh typing?

Problems in Rh typing fall into two main categories: the red cells react less strongly with the antiserum than the average cell, or the red cells react in the control procedure as well as in the test.

Unusually Weak Agglutination

Each of the common antigens of the Rh system has been found in a variant form. The variant form of D (D^u) has already been described. There are also variants of C, c, E and e, as well as individuals whose red cells show depression of all the Rh antigens. Descriptions of these variants may be found in other publications. In some cases the variant antigen may react with one antiserum of a given specificity and not with another of the same apparent specificity. This occurs because the two antisera are not in fact identical, although the difference between them is insignificant when testing the vast majority of blood samples.

Cells sensitized with anti-D *in vivo*, such as cells of babies with hemolytic disease due to anti-D, may not type correctly by any direct agglutination method because all or almost all D antigen sites may be blocked. When *all* the D antigen sites on the cells take up anti-D *in vivo*, no sites are available for the attachment of the anti-D in the reagent and the cells appear to be Rh negative. False negative tests due to such heavy sensitization are extremely rare. If an eluate prepared from sensitized red cells is shown to contain anti-D, the red cells are then established as Rh positive; were they really Rh negative, they would not have absorbed anti-D *in vivo* and eluates could not contain anti-D.

Positive Controls

The number of cells that cannot be correctly typed because of positive controls depends largely on the suspending medium used for the red cells being tested and whether the Rh antiserum is a low-protein or high-protein reagent. As discussed earlier, the use of saline-suspended cells and a low-protein antiserum minimizes false agglutination in Rh typing. The test situation in which false positive agglutination is most likely to be encountered is that in which a patient's red cells are suspended in his or her own serum and tested with a high-protein, potentiated Rh antiserum. The false agglutination is caused by abnormal proteins and/or autoantibodies in the patient's serum. The potentiator in the antiserum allows the red cells to approach one another more closely than they would in a saline environment and the ability of the autoagglutinin to cross-link the cells is thus enhanced. These problems can be readily resolved by washing the patient's cells free of serum, suspending them in saline, and retesting with either a low-protein or a high-protein reagent.

A less readily resolved problem in Rh typing may occur when the red cells being tested have a positive direct antiglobulin test. The extent of the problem depends on the Rh antiserum used. Some of these cells, especially those with a very strongly positive direct antiglobulin test, will react with Rh-hr Control, thereby invalidating a positive test result obtained with a high-protein anti-D reagent. Virtually all patients with a positive direct antiglobulin test can be typed accurately if a low-protein anti-D serum is used, and if the patient's cells are washed and suspended in saline. Because the test for D^u includes the antiglobulin procedure as its final phase, cells with a positive direct antiglobulin test, whether from a D^u positive or D^u negative individual, will give a positive test for D^u (as well as a positive D^u control). A patient whose cells are not agglutinated by anti-D but have a positive direct antiglobulin test (and therefore a positive D^u test) should receive only Rh negative blood. On the other hand, if donor blood reacts as D negative but the test for D^u and the direct antiglobulin test are positive, the blood should not be used.

4.4 QUESTIONS

Variant forms of the C, c, E and e antigens

☐ have

☐ have not

been found.

have

What problem in Rh typing may be caused by variant forms of Rh antigens (such as D^u)?

_____

**unusually weak
agglutination**

What problems in Rh typing may be caused by using a high-protein, potentiated Rh antiserum?

_____

**false positive results;
sticky buttons**

The problem of false positive results caused by high-protein, potentiated antisera can usually be resolved by washing the cells free of

serum and suspending them in _____ .

saline

A patient whose red cells type as D negative but are agglutinated in the test for D^u and who has a positive direct antiglobulin test should receive:

☐ D positive blood.

☐ D negative blood.

D negative blood.

Donor red cells which type as D negative but are agglutinated in the test for D^u and exhibit a positive direct antiglobulin test

☐ should

☐ should not

be used for transfusions.

should not

Chapter Five:
Antibody Detection

Objectives for Chapter Five

Upon completion of this chapter you should be able to:

5.1
- **Describe the uses of the following test procedures:**
  - antibody screening
  - crossmatching
  - reverse grouping

- **Explain the significance of alloantibodies and autoantibodies**

5.2
- **Describe the test procedures used to detect antibodies in transfusion candidates**

- **Describe the test procedures used to detect antibodies in prenatal patients**

- **Describe the test procedures used to detect antibodies in donor units**

5.1

What tests are used to detect antibodies?

Most blood group antibodies are found when testing the serum of an individual — in antibody screening, crossmatching, or reverse grouping. Most antibodies are found in the absence of the corresponding antigen and they are called **alloantibodies**. Occasionally antibodies may be detected bound to red cells *in vivo*, either alone or in addition to circulating antibodies. As described in Focus Question 1.6, antibody bound to red cells is demonstrated in the direct antiglobulin test. When properly performed, a positive direct antiglobulin test denotes the presence of antigen and the corresponding antibody in the same individual, indicating either an autoimmune state, an incompatible transfusion, or hemolytic disease of the newborn. It is essential to distinguish autoantibodies found in autoimmune states from alloantibodies found in transfusion reactions and hemolytic disease of the newborn.

The choice of procedures and red cells for antibody detection tests depends on the purpose of the test. As explained in Focus Question 3.2, reverse grouping is intended to demonstrate the expected antibodies anti-A and anti-B. The procedure is a simple one using A_1 and B red cells suspended in saline and is performed at room temperature. Although these conditions are suitable for anti-A and anti-B, they are not adequate for the detection of clinically significant antibodies that react optimally at 37°C. The purpose of antibody screening tests — to detect unexpected antibodies that may cause *in vivo* destruction of red cells — is best served by more extensive testing. The individual being tested also affects the decision as to how antibody screening tests are done. For example, an antibody in a prenatal patient or a blood donor may not be as dangerous as the same antibody in a transfusion candidate.

5.1 QUESTIONS

Antibodies found in the absence of the corresponding antigen are

called _____ .

A positive direct antiglobulin test denotes the presence of:

☐ antibody in serum.

☐ antibody on red cells.

Autoantibodies indicate _____ states.

A positive direct antiglobulin test due to alloantibodies may be found

in _____

and _____ .

Match the following:

1 ____ expected anti-A and   A   reverse grouping
       anti-B

2 ____ unexpected antibodies   B   antibody screening

---

alloantibodies

antibody on red cells.

autoimmune

transfusion reactions

**hemolytic disease of
the newborn**

1 A

2 B

5.2

What is the importance of antibody detection?

Transfusion Candidates

There is a potential danger for a patient whose serum contains blood group antibodies if he or she receives a transfusion of any red cells except his or her own. If an antibody capable of destroying red cells is not detected prior to transfusion and incompatible red cells are given, the consequences could be serious, even fatal. Because of the risk involved, two procedures to detect antibodies are recommended for any patient who is likely to require blood in the immediate future: an antibody screening test and a crossmatch.* Similar methods are used, but the two tests will not necessarily detect the same antibody because of differences between the antigen make-up of reagent red cells and the red cells of prospective donors.

The most sensitive antibody screening test is one using reagent red cells obtained from two or three different individuals and processed separately. The screening test is less sensitive if the cells are pooled together. With separate cell samples, the user is assured that there is no dilution of antigens which could cause a weak antibody to go undetected. The selection of cells homozygous for certain antigens also enhances the sensitivity of the test system. Antibodies such as anti-c, anti-Jk^a and anti-M frequently react better with homozygous cells than with heterozygous cells and in some cases they are detected only when homozygous cells are used. Antibodies that react more strongly with homozygous than with heterozygous cells are said to show "dosage."

Use of various test conditions is an additional means of enhancing the sensitivity of an antibody screening test. Room temperature tests are not essential; if performed, they should be centrifuged immediately and not be allowed to stand. Incubation at 37°C is essential because an antibody which sensitizes or agglutinates red cells *in vitro* at 37°C will probably destroy incompatible red cells *in vivo*. Prior to the antiglobulin procedure, tests can be incubated in saline, albumin or low ionic strength solution. Since each medium provides conditions that are optimal for certain antibodies, the use of more than one method is desirable. IgM antibodies usually agglutinate red cells in saline. Some IgG antibodies (especially those with Rh specificity) agglutinate red cells in albumin; other IgG molecules do not cause agglutination but only sensitize red cells in saline, albumin or low ionic strength solution. The major difference among the saline, albumin and low ionic media is the rate at which antibody uptake occurs.

---

*This test is variously referred to as the crossmatch, the compatibility test, or the test for serological incompatibility.

For maximum sensitivity in antibody detection, polyspecific anti-human serum is required. As discussed in Focus Question 1.6, this reagent recognizes IgG and complement; *in vivo* red blood cell destruction can result from either sensitization by IgG or complement fixed to the cell by the action of IgG or IgM antibodies.

In most cases, a test of the patient's serum with the red cells of every prospective donor is performed prior to transfusion. Exceptions may be made, particularly in life-threatening emergencies. The principle of this test is the same as the antibody screening test but the red cells are those of prospective donors rather than reagent red cells. Usually the ABO group and Rh type are all that is known about the donor's cells. However, if the transfusion candidate is known to have an antibody, donor units which lack the corresponding antigen should have been preselected by testing them with antiserum of the appropriate specificity. Preselection of donor units does not eliminate the need for crossmatching because this serves as a check on errors in ABO grouping as well as a means of detecting unexpected antibodies. If the antibody is a very uncommon one and an alternative example is unavailable or limited in quantity, the patient's serum should be used to select apparently compatible donors or donor units. If possible, the donor blood should then be tested with the rare serum to assure that it lacks the antigen.

Prenatal Patients

To predict the likelihood of hemolytic disease of the newborn, all prenatal patients should have at least one antibody screening test and preferably more than one. Any IgG antibody, regardless of specificity, can cross the placenta and has the potential to destroy the red cells of the fetus. The extent of cell destruction depends on the level (titer) of the antibody, as well as the presence of the antigen on the fetal cells. If the most sensitive antibody screening test is desired, the patient's serum should be tested with screening cells from at least two individual donors. When additional tests can be performed during pregnancy, a less sensitive but more economical method using pooled screening cells may be acceptable.

Once an antibody has been detected in a prenatal patient, it must be identified, not only to anticipate hemolytic disease of the newborn, but also to determine whether Rh immune globulin is indicated.

Either polyspecific anti-human serum or monospecific anti-IgG will detect IgG antibody in the maternal serum. For a number of reasons, complement is less significant in prenatal screening than in a transfusion situation.

- In many cases prenatal blood samples are mailed to the testing laboratory and, as a result, they are deficient in complement.

- Most of the antibodies which require complement for their detection are IgM, and IgM does not cross the placenta.

- Occasionally, an IgG antibody fixes complement and is detectable only by the anti-complement in polyspecific anti-human serum. Because complement levels in the fetus are low, such an antibody is not likely to cause hemolytic disease of the newborn.

Detection of an antibody in a prenatal patient can serve as an early warning of possible difficulty in obtaining compatible blood should the patient ever need transfusion. In that event, the antibody screening test would be repeated and a crossmatch would also be done. The use of polyspecific anti-human serum is advocated for pretransfusion tests.

Donor Units

Simpler and less sensitive methods than those used to detect antibodies in patients are acceptable for donor screening. Experience has shown that no harm results if blood or plasma containing a weak antibody is infused, undoubtedly because it is diluted in the patient's circulation. In many laboratories each unit of plasma is tested with a pool of two screening cells at 37°C by the antiglobulin technique. No one individual can provide red cells with all the clinically significant antigens. Ideally, at least one of the two donors contributing to the pool would be homozygous for antigens such as c, E, M and Jk^a. Polyspecific anti-human serum is used for donor screening in some institutions; others prefer anti-IgG serum. Either reagent is acceptable because, in most cases, plasma is tested rather than serum. Complement is inactive in plasma. Some workers use an enzyme method for donor screening. The fact that there are only a few reports of transfusion reactions due to antibodies in donor units might imply that donor screening is unnecessary. However, there are other factors to be considered.

- Rh negative blood is sometimes given to an Rh positive person, especially in an emergency. If the unit were to contain anti-D, the patient could develop a positive direct antiglobulin test which could be confusing on subsequent testing.

- If an obstetrical patient were to receive a unit of blood containing anti-D, there would be no way of knowing that the antibody was passive and not actively produced by the patient. Under such circumstances Rh immune globulin might be withheld erroneously.

- The donor may be a patient someday. Knowing that he or she is immunized and knowing the specificity of the antibody are important for the donor's welfare.

- Donor units can be a source of antibodies for use as reagents. They may be supplied to antiserum manufacturers or frozen for use in the laboratory where they were found.

5.2 QUESTIONS

What test(s) is (are) recommended for any patient about to receive a blood transfusion?

antibody screening test and a test for serological incompatibility (crossmatch)

_____

_____

Which type of antibody screening test is the most sensitive?

one using cells obtained from two or three different individuals

☐ one using cells obtained from two or three different individuals

☐ one using a pool of cells

The selection of

homozygous

☐ homozygous

☐ heterozygous

cells enhances the sensitivity of the test system for certain antibodies.

Antibodies which react more strongly with homozygous than with heterozygous cells are said to:

☐ be "inconsistent."

show "dosage."

☐ show "dosage."

Match the following:

1   B

1 _____ IgG antibodies

A   usually agglutinate red cells in saline

2   A

2 _____ IgM antibodies

B   depending on their specificity, may sensitize red cells in saline, albumin or low ionic strength solution

It is essential to perform antibody tests at

☐ room temperature

37°C

☐ 37°C

because an antibody that reacts at this temperature is most

destroy incompatible red cells

likely to _____

_____ _in vivo._

	The use of polyspecific anti-human serum provides for maximum sensitivity in antibody detection since it will recognize _____
IgG	
complement	and _____ .
	If a transfusion candidate is known to have an antibody, donor units are preselected
	☐ for
to avoid	☐ to avoid
	the presence of the corresponding antigen.
	Preselection of donor units
	☐ eliminates
does not eliminate	☐ does not eliminate
	the need for crossmatching.
	If the patient's serum contains a rare antibody and a reagent serum of
the patient's	the same specificity is unavailable, _____ serum may be used to select apparently compatible donors.
	Which antibody class has the potential to cross the placenta?
	☐ IgM
IgG	☐ IgG
	In hemolytic disease of the newborn the extent of red cell destruction depends on the presence of the antigen on the fetal cells and on the
level (titer)	_____ of the antibody.
	In prenatal screening, complement is
	☐ less important
less important	☐ more important
	than in a transfusion situation.

When testing for the presence of antibodies in donor units,

☐ less

☐ more

sensitive tests are acceptable than when testing the patient's serum for antibodies.

Antibodies present in donor units

☐ frequently

☐ rarely

cause transfusion reactions.

less

rarely

Chapter Six:

Antibody Identification

Objectives for Chapter Six

Upon completion of this chapter you should be able to:

6.1 • **Explain the importance of antibody identification in:**
  • transfusion candidates
  • obstetrical patients
  • donors

6.2 • **Describe the tests used to identify antibodies**

• **Discuss the significance of grading reactions in antibody identification**

• **Explain the use of auto controls in antibody identification**

• **Describe the use of an ANTIGRAM Antigen Profile in antibody identification**

• **Discuss the relative frequency with which different antibodies are found**

6.3 • **Discuss the confidence limits which should be established in antibody identification**

6.1

Why is it important to identify the specificity of antibodies?

The significance of a given specificity differs depending on whether the serum is from a transfusion candidate, an obstetrical patient or a donor. The many reasons to identify antibodies in each group follow:

Transfusion Candidates

- To select the appropriate antisera to type the donor red cells in addition to performing the crossmatch

- To characterize the serum completely — the presence of more than one antibody may not be obvious when using only two or three screening cells

- To be prepared should blood be needed in an emergency

- To have a record of the identity of the antibody should the antibody drop in titer to an undetectable level

- To aid in the identification of antibodies produced at a later time

Obstetrical Patients

- To evaluate the need and be prepared for an exchange transfusion of the newborn:

  - Blood for an exchange transfusion should be shown to be negative for the corresponding antigen as well as crossmatch-compatible with the mother's serum.

  - If compatible blood proves to be rare, time is needed to find a suitable donor.

  - Additional antibodies may have developed late in pregnancy and repeating the identification will assure their detection.

- To evaluate the need for Rh immune globulin:

  - An Rh negative woman should receive Rh immune globulin if the antibody in her serum is other than anti-D and if the baby is D or D^u positive.

- To test the father for the corresponding antigen and determine his zygosity

- To be prepared should the mother need blood

- To evaluate the need for amniocentesis:

  — Amniocentesis is the procedure in which a needle is inserted through the abdominal wall into the amnionic sac. **Amnionic fluid** can be aspirated and results of tests on this fluid for bilirubin can be used to monitor the degree of hemolysis in the fetus of an immunized woman. The specificity of the maternal antibody and its titer are significant factors which affect the decision to perform amniocentesis.

  — The indication for amniocentesis is the finding of anti-D or another antibody known to cause hemolytic disease of the newborn. An antiglobulin titer of 16 is the usual level above which amniocentesis is performed; however, this level should be established by each laboratory depending on the methods used for titration of antibodies.

  — Amnionic fluid should not be monitored if the antibody is identified as one which does not cause hemolytic disease of the newborn, most notably anti-Le^a or anti-Le^b.

  — Amniocentesis should not be performed if the antibody has been produced as a result of transfusion and the baby could not have the corresponding antigen as shown by testing the father.

Donors

- To avoid the confusion that can result from passively infused antibodies (usually they are not clinically dangerous)

- To inform the donor that he or she is immunized

- To make use of the antibody in testing other donors or patients, or for educational purposes

6.1 QUESTIONS

Once antibodies have been detected in transfusion candidates it

☐ is

☐ is not

important to identify the specificity of the antibodies.

The identification of antibodies in transfusion candidates is required:

☐ to select the appropriate antisera to type the donor red cells.

☐ to be prepared for an emergency transfusion.

☐ both of the above

In which obstetrical situation(s) should amnionic fluid be monitored?

☐ when the antibody is identified as anti-Le^a or anti-Le^b

☐ when the antibody is one that is known to cause hemolytic disease of the newborn and the titer is 16 or greater

Donor antibodies should be identified to avoid:

☐ the confusion that passively infused antibodies can cause.

☐ dangerous hemolytic reactions which can threaten the patient's life.

---

is

both of the above

when the antibody is one that is known to cause hemolytic disease of the newborn and the titer is 16 or greater

the confusion that passively infused antibodies can cause.

6.2

How are antibodies identified?

Whereas the exact methods for performing antibody identification will be found in the package inserts for reagent red blood cells, the principles involved in developing the methodology for antibody identification are discussed here.

Knowledge of the identity and serological characteristics of an antibody contribute to the evaluation of its clinical significance. In order to characterize the antibody or antibodies and to aid in their identification, testing is performed at various temperatures and in different media. The method to be used for identification should be selected on the basis of the mode of optimum reactivity observed in detection procedures. However, even if reactions were observed only in the antiglobulin phase of screening, each step of the identification procedure should be completed, read and recorded. Time is rarely saved by taking shortcuts in antibody identification. Antibody identification should include testing the serum with a panel of cells using at least one of the currently available enhancement media as well as the antiglobulin test. Albumin is especially useful in antibody identification because it potentiates agglutination of red cells at 37°C, especially when Rh antibodies are present.

Whereas deliberately screening for cold agglutinins is discouraged, their presence is indicated if the strength of the reaction weakens as the temperature is raised or if the agglutination in the antiglobulin phase is weaker than that observed at 37°C. Under these circumstances the panel should be tested in duplicate. One panel should be set up without additives and first incubated at room temperature followed by 18°C; the other one with an enhancement medium added is incubated at 37°C and followed by the antiglobulin procedure.

For antibody identification tests to be meaningful, the results of each step of the procedure should be read carefully for hemolysis and/or agglutination and noted on the recording sheet. There are two important reasons to record the strength of reactions. First, variation in strength may be the only indication of a mixture of antibodies. Second, observation of stronger reactions with homozygous than with heterozygous cells (dosage) adds a dimension to the identification which would otherwise be based only on positive and negative reactions. Since grading the strength of agglutination is subjective, it is necessary to standardize the system used within each laboratory so that the strength of reactions recorded can be correctly interpreted by any member of the staff.

The first step in interpreting any panel is to note the **autologous** control. The "auto" control is a test of the patient's serum with the patient's cells treated in the same manner as all other cells of the panel. To be most meaningful, the patient's cells should be suspended in the same diluent as the cells of the panel. Even though an auto control has been run as a part of antibody detection, it should be repeated with each panel. If the auto control is negative, it serves as a nonreactive cell for comparison with other cells of the panel. This is especially valuable if some cells of the panel are very weakly agglutinated. If the auto control is positive, one can compare the strength of reaction of the patient's serum with his or her own cells to reactions with cells of the panel at different temperatures and in different media.

Regardless of which combination of methods is used, a single antibody is usually not difficult to identify. The identification is accomplished by matching the pattern of reactions of the test results against the patterns displayed on the ANTIGRAM Antigen Profile. Observing the medium in which the reaction was most strongly demonstrated aids in locating the pattern on the ANTIGRAM and if the antibody is reacting typically, aids in its identification. The pattern of reactions, however, not the medium or temperature of the reactions, defines specificity. Whereas antibodies of a certain specificity usually react optimally in a certain medium or at a characteristic temperature, there are many exceptions.

When a single antibody is present, the specificity revealed by the pattern formed by the positive reactions is usually quite obvious. But before drawing a final conclusion it must be determined that no other pattern or combination of patterns could also match that of the unknown. (In well-prepared panels overlapping patterns within a group which typically exhibit similar reactivity are rare; however, it is not possible to prevent all overlapping patterns.) To rule out additional antibodies, note (cross out) the antigens that are present on the cells of the panel that were not agglutinated by the patient's serum. If all significant antigens are crossed out except the one corresponding to the antibody already selected, the specificity is confirmed and it is unlikely there is a second antibody. An example of how to use the ANTIGRAM Antigen Profile to identify a single antibody and establish that no other antibodies are present is shown in Table 6.2A.

To prevent drawing false conclusions, only antigens that are expressed as homozygotes should be crossed out. Otherwise, antibodies that show such pronounced dosage as to be nonreactive with heterozygous cells will be falsely excluded. An example of this possibility is illustrated in Table 6.2B.

After tentative identification has been made, confirmation should include testing the patient's cells for the corresponding antigen. This can be done using either a commercial antiserum or antibodies of the same specificity saved from other problem cases of the same ABO group.

As has been discussed previously, certain antibodies are produced more commonly than others. This is due to the relative immunogenicity of the antigen and the percentage of persons lacking the antigen, as well as the frequency, quantity and route of introduction of the immunogen. Table 6.2C has been constructed on the basis of a review of the literature. The exact order of frequency with which different antibodies are detected varies from one study to another, depending on whether patients or donors were the predominant population considered in the report. Hospital patients are older, on the average, and may have had repeated exposure to many red cell antigens by way of transfusions or pregnancies, while donors are less likely to be immunized. Furthermore, some reports are from reference laboratories and the expertise or interest of that particular laboratory affects the material sent to them for study. The likelihood of finding certain antibodies will also depend on the manner of testing. Extended room temperature incubation, used commonly in the past, increased the number of cold antibodies reported in some studies, and the routine use of enzymes increased the number of anti-E and antibodies of the Lewis system in others. Table 6.2C does not include anti-I or anti-IH even though they were among the most common antibodies observed prior to the elimination of room temperature incubation for antibody detection tests. Anti-I and anti-IH are cold autoantibodies of no clinical significance except in the very rare condition of cold agglutinin disease when anti-I may cause *in vivo* hemolysis if the patient becomes chilled.

Table 6.2A In this table the patient's serum (shown on the right) reacts with cells 2, 3, 5, 6, 8 and 9 when tested with anti-human serum and fails to react with cells 1, 4, 7 and 10. This pattern matches that in the column labeled Fy^a; therefore, the antibody present in this patient's serum is probably anti-Fy^a. To be sure that no other antibody is present, note (i.e., cross out) the antigens present on the cells that did not react with the patient's serum. The patient's serum did not react with cell 1, and cell 1 is D+, C+, e+, k+, Fy(b+), Jk(b+), s+, and M+. Had the patient's serum contained an antibody to any of these antigens, cell 1 would have been agglutinated. Therefore, the probability that any of these antibodies is present but masked by the reactions of the anti-Fy^a is excluded. The same can be done for cells 4, 7 and 10. Since all antigens on this panel (other than Fy^a) are present on at least one of the nonreactive cells, it is unlikely that any additional antibody is present.

Cell No.	Rh-hr					KELL		DUFFY		KIDD		MNS				Patient's Serum		
	D	C	E	c	e	K	k	Fy^a	Fy^b	Jk^a	Jk^b	S	s	M	N	Cell No.	37° Alb	AHS
1	+	+	o	o	+	o	+	o	+	o	+	o	+	+	o	1	0	0
2	+	+	o	o	+	+	+	+	o	o	+	+	+	o	+	2	0	4+
3	+	o	+	+	o	o	+	+	+	+	o	o	+	o	+	3	0	4+
4	+	o	o	+	+	o	+	o	o	+	o	+	+	o	+	4	0	0
5	o	+	o	+	+	o	+	+	+	+	o	+	+	+	o	5	0	4+
6	o	o	+	+	+	o	+	+	o	+	o	+	+	+	+	6	0	4+
7	o	o	o	+	+	+	+	o	+	+	o	o	+	+	o	7	0	0
8	o	o	o	+	+	o	+	+	o	o	+	o	+	o	+	8	0	4+
9	o	o	o	+	+	+	+	+	+	+	+	+	o	+	o	9	0	4+
10	+	o	+	+	+	o	+	o	+	+	+	+	o	+	+	10	0	0
11	Auto Control															11	0	0

Table 6.2B In this example the pattern of reactions of the patient's serum matches that of anti-Jk^a. Note the weaker reactions (dosage effect) with cells 4 and 6 compared to cell 2. They are heterozygous Jk(a+b+) while cell 2 is homozygous Jk(a+b-). To show that no other antibodies are present, note the antigens present on cell 1, which is nonreactive with the patient's serum — k, Fy^a, Fy^b, Jk^b, S, s and M. However, Fy^a, Fy^b, S and s should not be crossed out because they are all heterozygous. Cell 3 eliminates Fy^a and N while cell 5 eliminates Fy^b and s. None of the non-reactive cells is homozygous S (S+s-); therefore, if S were crossed out based on cell 1, anti-S showing dosage might be falsely excluded. A complete panel of 10 or 12 cells would probably contain cells that are Jk(a-) and S+s-, and exclude the probability that anti-S is present but masked by the anti-Jk^a. (Homozygous K+ cells are very rare. Anti-K is usually excluded based on a heterozygous cell, but anti-K does not characteristically show dosage.)

Cell No.	KELL		DUFFY		KIDD		MNS				Patient's Serum		
	K	k	Fy^a	Fy^b	Jk^a	Jk^b	S	s	M	N	Cell No.	37° Alb	AHS
1	o	+	+	+	o	+	+	+	+	o	1	0	0
2	+	+	o	+	+	o	o	+	o	+	2	0	4+
3	+	+	+	o	o	+	+	+	o	+	3	0	0
4	o	+	o	o	+	+	+	o	+	+	4	0	2+
5	o	+	o	+	o	+	o	+	+	+	5	0	0
6	o	+	+	+	+	+	o	+	+	+	6	0	2+

Table 6.2C The antibodies are grouped in the approximate order of frequency found — the group at the top being the most common and the group at the bottom rare. Antibodies not listed are extremely rare. The likelihood of finding antibodies to low frequency antigens will vary depending on the antigens supplied as reagent red cells.

anti-D with or without anti-C or anti-E	
anti-Le^a and anti-Le^b — alone or together	
anti-K	
anti-E	anti-P$_1$
anti-c	anti-cE
anti-Fy^a	anti-M
anti-Jk^a	anti-S
anti-Ce	anti-e
anti-Jk^b	anti-N
anti-s	anti-Fy^b

6.2 QUESTIONS

Antibody identification tests should be performed:

☐ at various temperatures and in different media.

☐ at one specific temperature and in an appropriate medium.

Evaluation of the clinical significance of an antibody is dependent upon

_____

and _____ .

When the presence of a cold agglutinin is indicated, one test panel without additives should be performed at

_____

and a second panel with additives at

_____ .

Variation in the strength of agglutination may be an indication of

_____

or _____ .

Noting the autologous control is the

☐ first

☐ last

step in interpreting any panel.

If an autologous control has been run as part of antibody detection, it is

☐ advisable

☐ not necessary

to include an autologous control with the identification panel.

Sidebar (answers):

at various temperatures and in different media.

the specificity of the anti-body
its serological characteristics

room temperature and 18°C

37°C

a mixture of antibodies

an antibody showing dosage

first

advisable

In the case of alloantibodies, the auto control should be:

☐ positive.

☐ negative.

negative.

To identify an antibody, the pattern of reactions of test results is read against the pattern displayed on a(n)

ANTIGRAM Antigen Profile

_____ .

To rule out additional antibodies when interpreting the results of an antibody panel, the antigens present on the

☐ reactive

☐ nonreactive

nonreactive

cells are crossed out.

When matching the pattern of reactions, only nonreactive cells:

☐ heterozygous

☐ homozygous

homozygous

for a particular antigen should be crossed out.

The frequency with which different antibodies are produced depends upon:

☐ immunogenicity.

☐ the percentage of persons lacking the antigen.

☐ frequency, quantity, and route of introduction.

all the above

☐ all the above

Anti-I and anti-IH are

☐ rarely

rarely

☐ frequently

clinically significant.

6.3

Is it possible to draw the wrong conclusion in antibody identification?

Chance alone could account for the pattern of reactions observed with a panel of reagent red blood cells. A 95 percent confidence level is considered adequate in antibody identification; that is, a probability of one in twenty that chance alone accounts for the observed pattern. Provided three positive cells react and three negative cells do not react, this probability is established. If only two cells are positive and they react, five negative cells must be nonreactive. If only one cell is positive, 19 must be negative in order to establish identity with the 95 percent level of confidence. A seven- or eight-cell panel might be adequate if we dealt with single antibodies only, and if the pattern of cells of a panel were ideal in that there were no patterns which overlapped or were masked. However, mixtures of antibodies are not uncommon and the distribution of antigens in the population makes it essentially impossible to provide a suitable panel with fewer than 10 to 12 cells. If the number of test cells available does not give this confidence level, other procedures should be used to confirm the presumed identity of the antibody; e.g., neutralization with substance or destruction of the antigen by enzyme treatment.

If the pattern of reaction is not that of a single common antibody, it is best to assume that the reactions are due to a mixture of common antibodies before looking for some exotic single specificity. Simple mixtures of antibodies are usually not difficult to identify if one keeps in mind that the mixture is likely to be a combination of those antibodies that are often found as single antibodies. For example, in Rh negative people, anti-D will often be accompanied by anti-K, anti-Fy^a or anti-P$_1$. There is one important exception to this assumption: anti-C is extremely rare as a single antibody and yet it is commonly found in the same serum with anti-D. In Rh positive persons common combinations are anti-E plus anti-K; anti-K plus anti-Fy^a; anti-E plus anti-Fy^a; anti-c plus anti-K, etc.

Even though a single antibody or a simple mixture of antibodies should be easily identifiable, there are many factors that introduce confusion:

- Antibodies of a given specificity do not always react as expected, i.e., in the same medium or at the same temperature as most others of the same specificity.

- A single antibody showing dosage may appear to be a mixture of antibodies.

- Very weak antibodies may not react with all cells that carry the antigen, especially if the antibody shows dosage or if the antigen varies in strength (as is typical of anti-P_1).

- Complex mixtures of antibodies are rarely easy to identify.

For a more complete discussion of problems encountered in antibody identification including discussions of autoantibodies, the reader is referred to the publications listed in Sources of Additional Information in the back of this book.

6.3 QUESTIONS

What confidence level is considered adequate in antibody testing?

☐ 95 percent

☐ 99 percent

Which of the following would establish such a confidence level?

☐ three positive cells react and three negative cells do not react

☐ two positive cells react and four negative cells do not react

☐ one positive cell reacts and nine negative cells do not react

Because of the distribution of antigens and the common occurrence of mixtures of antibodies, it is essentially impossible to provide a suitable panel with fewer than:

☐ 8 cells.

☐ 10 to 12 cells.

If the pattern of reactions is not that of a single common antibody, it is most likely due to:

☐ a single rare antibody.

☐ a mixture of common antibodies.

Which of the following statements is true?

☐ Anti-C is commonly found in the same serum as anti-D.

☐ Anti-C is commonly found as a single antibody.

Antibodies showing dosage may appear to be

_____ .

Complex mixtures of antibodies are

☐ usually

☐ rarely

easy to identify.

---

95 percent

three positive cells react and three negative cells do not react

10 to 12 cells.

a mixture of common antibodies.

Anti-C is commonly found in the same serum as anti-D.

a mixture of antibodies

rarely

Chapter Seven:

Blood Group Antibodies Other Than ABO

Objectives for Chapter Seven

Upon completion of this chapter you should be able to:

7.1 • **Name the antibodies which are most frequently found in patients and donors**

7.2 • **Describe the clinical significance and *in vitro* characteristics of anti-D**

7.3 • **Describe the clinical significance and *in vitro* characteristics of anti-Le^a and anti-Le^b**

7.4 • **Describe the clinical significance and *in vitro* characteristics of anti-K**

7.5 • **Describe the clinical significance and *in vitro* characteristics of anti-Fy^a**

7.6 • **Describe the clinical significance and *in vitro* characteristics of anti-Jk^a and anti-Jk^b**

7.7 • **Describe the clinical significance and *in vitro* characteristics of anti-M**

• **Describe the clinical significance and *in vitro* characteristics of anti-S**

7.8 • **Describe the clinical significance and *in vitro* characteristics of anti-P$_1$**

7.1

Which antibodies are most likely to be found in patients and donors?

Some antibodies are found far more frequently than others due to (1) the frequency of antigens in the population, (2) the ability of the antigen to stimulate antibody production, that is, whether or not it is an effective immunogen and (3) the presence of non-human sources of antigen similar to blood group antigens. These natural substances stimulate the production of antibodies even in persons who have not been exposed to red blood cells. The most common alloantibodies found are shown in Table 6.2C in decreasing order of their incidence. These antibodies will be discussed in sufficient detail to alert the technologist to the basic significance of each antibody. Further details of all blood group systems abound in other texts listed in Sources of Additional Information at the end of the book. Rare antibodies will not be covered here unless mentioned as part of a system already under discussion.

Each focus question will discuss a commonly found antibody and other antibodies of the same system. The clinical significance of the antibodies will be described for transfusion candidates, for obstetrical patients and for blood donors. Throughout this chapter it is recommended that donor units which are found to have antibodies should be used as Red Blood Cells. (Red Blood Cells will be capitalized when referring to the component remaining after removal of most of the plasma from sedimented or centrifuged whole blood.) There is very little evidence that antibodies passively transfused to a patient will cause any red blood cell destruction. Most donor centers continue to screen for antibodies to avoid the confusion created by passively infused antibodies, but room temperature testing is being deemphasized. The *in vitro* characteristics of the antibodies are summarized in table format to allow easy reference or review by the blood bank technologist. The properties of the corresponding antigens are described. Finally, other significant or interesting points relative to the antibodies or the genetics of the blood group system are discussed.

7.2

Which are the significant antibodies of the Rh system?

Anti-D is the most important antibody of the Rh system. Its clinical significance and *in vitro* characteristics are described in this focus question. A discussion of the immunogenicity of the D antigen and a brief discussion of other antibodies of the Rh system are also included.

Clinical Significance

For transfusion candidates. Whereas anti-D is one of the most common antibodies found in transfusion candidates, it is not usually a cause of transfusion reactions. This is because of the universal practice of giving Rh negative blood to Rh negative patients. A transfusion reaction due to anti-D presupposes two errors — failing to detect the antibody and mistyping the donor. If a transfusion accident does occur due to Rh incompatibility, the reaction is extravascular and the severity depends on the many conditions discussed in Focus Question 8.2.

For obstetrical patients. Hemolytic disease of the newborn due to anti-D is becoming a rare occurrence. However, in spite of the introduction of Rh immune globulin in 1968, the disease has not been eradicated. Most cases of hemolytic disease of the newborn seen today are due to ABO incompatibility, but this disease is usually mild. Anti-D remains the most common cause of severe hemolytic disease of the newborn. For a more complete description of hemolytic disease of the newborn, see Focus Questions 8.4 and 8.5.

For donors. The most significant antibody found in a donor population is anti-D. Anti-D in a donor unit will not harm the Rh negative recipient of the blood, but confusion may be created. For example, when the serum of a recently transfused patient contains anti-D, it is assumed that the antibody was produced by the patient. If this were an obstetrical patient at term, Rh immune globulin might be withheld. As a second example, a positive direct antiglobulin test can result when D negative blood with anti-D is given to an Rh positive patient in an emergency. Subsequent serological investigation of the patient could be quite confusing.

In Vitro Characteristics

The *in vitro* characteristics of anti-D are summarized in the following table.

The *In Vitro* Characteristics of Anti-D
• Is detected by the antiglobulin test
• Demonstrates agglutination in the presence of bovine serum albumin or with enzyme-treated cells
• Is rarely reactive at or below room temperature
• Shows variability in strength of reaction with cells of different genotypes, but does not show dosage

D as an Immunogen

D is probably the most effective immunogen of all red blood cell antigens. More than one-half of all Rh negative people will produce anti-D if transfused with D positive blood.

Other Antibodies

Among Rh negative people, anti-C is a common antibody but it is almost always found with anti-D and its potential significance is masked by the anti-D. Anti-E is also found frequently with anti-D in Rh negative people.

Among Rh positive patients, anti-E is by far the most common Rh antibody, but anti-c (hr′) is more significant. About 51 percent of Rh positive people can produce anti-E alone and 18 percent can produce anti-c alone or in combination with anti-E. Anti-E is often a saline agglutinin (IgM) and rarely causes hemolytic disease of the newborn; however, a patient whose serum contains anti-E must receive E negative blood. Anti-c, on the other hand, is usually IgG and can cause transfusion reactions and hemolytic disease of the newborn. Anti-C in an Rh positive person (DcE or Dce) is very rare.

Anti-e, a common autoantibody, is not often found as an alloantibody. There are two reasons for this: (1) less than two percent of Rh positive people are e negative and (2) e is a very weak immunogen. Of interest, however, is the fact that the e antigen has many variant forms and a single example of anti-e may not react with all cells found to be e positive when tested with another example of anti-e.

7.3

Which are the significant antibodies of the Lewis system?

The most important antibodies of the Lewis system are anti-Le^a and anti-Le^b. The clinical significance and *in vitro* characteristics of these two antibodies are described in this focus question. The immunogenicity of Le^a and Le^b and points to be kept in mind when identifying Lewis antibodies are also briefly discussed.

Clinical Significance

For transfusion candidates. Either anti-Le^a, anti-Le^b, or both may be found in a person who has never been exposed to red blood cells. Anti-Le^a is potentially hemolytic and patients with anti-Le^a should be given only Le(a–) blood. This presents no major problem since four out of five donors are Le(a–). Anti-Le^b can usually be ignored when found in a transfusion candidate. However, on rare occasions the antibody will agglutinate Le(b+) cells at 30°C or higher, or the antibody will react in the antiglobulin test using a prewarming technique. Only Le(b–) blood should be given under these circumstances.

For obstetrical patients. Anti-Le^a and anti-Le^b are found in obstetrical patients more often than would be expected. This is because during pregnancy Le^a and Le^b antigens are lost from the red cells. However, there are no substantiated cases of hemolytic disease of the newborn due to either anti-Le^a or anti-Le^b. The antibodies are usually IgM and cannot cross the placenta. When the occasional IgG antibody of Lewis specificity is present and crosses the placenta, there are Lewis substances throughout the body fluids of the baby which neutralize the antibody or antibodies. In addition, regardless of their Lewis genotype, the red blood cells of all newborns are Le(a–b–) and will not be affected by the antibody.

For donors. Antibodies of the Lewis system transfused to an Le(a+) or Le(b+) person will be neutralized by Lewis substances in the plasma of the recipient and will cause no harm.

In Vitro Characteristics

The *in vitro* characteristics of anti-Le^a and anti-Le^b are described in the following table.

The *In Vitro* Characteristics of Anti-Le^a and Anti-Le^b

Anti-Le^a

- Reacts in saline, albumin and/or by the antiglobulin technique

- Reacts over a wide temperature range

- May hemolyze Le(a+) red cells if serum is fresh

- Is neutralized by ORTHO Lewis Blood Group Substance

- Producer of the antibody is Le(a–b–) and need not have had prior exposure to red blood cells

Anti-Le^b

- Reacts in saline, albumin and/or by the antiglobulin technique

- The reactions are enhanced using enzyme-treated cells

- Is neutralized by ORTHO Lewis Blood Group Substance

- Producer of the antibody is almost always Le(a–b–) and need not have had prior exposure to red blood cells

---

Le^a and Le^b as Immunogens

Exposure to red blood cells is not a prerequisite for finding anti-Le^a and/or anti-Le^b in the serum of any person.

Antibodies of the Lewis system are very common and may require many hours of work to identify, but rarely are of any clinical significance. Omitting room temperature testing in antibody screening will significantly reduce the number of Lewis antibodies found. When detected, the fastest way to identify anti-Le^b, or anti-Le^a and anti-Le^b is to neutralize with ORTHO Lewis Blood Group Substance. Not only does this procedure identify the antibody but it also provides serum that can be used in additional tests to identify or exclude other antibodies.

7.4

Which are the significant antibodies of the Kell system?

Anti-K is the most important of the antibodies of the Kell system. Its clinical significance and *in vitro* characteristics are described below. In addition, the genetics of the Kell system and other antibodies of the Kell system are discussed briefly.

Clinical Significance

For transfusion candidates. Anti-K is one of the most common antibodies found either alone or in combination with other antibodies. It can be the cause of transfusion reactions if K positive donor red cells are accidentally given to a patient with anti-K. The reaction is extravascular, similar to that of any IgG antibody that characteristically does not fix complement.

For obstetrical patients. Anti-K can cause hemolytic disease of the newborn if the baby is K positive. The antibody in an obstetrical patient is not necessarily a cause for alarm but should be carefully investigated. The antibody in the mother may have been stimulated by transfused red cells and is of no concern, provided the baby is K negative. Testing the father of the baby and obtaining a careful transfusion history of the mother are especially important when anti-K is found in an obstetrical patient. Even if the father is K positive (only 9 percent of random persons are) he is probably heterozygous (97 percent of K positive persons are K/k) and the child has a 50 percent chance of being K negative and therefore unaffected by the antibody.

For donors. There is at least one documented case of passively acquired anti-K causing a transfusion reaction. Subsequently infused K positive donor red cells were destroyed by the antibody. Most antibodies in donors can be ignored if the plasma is removed and the cells are used as Red Blood Cells. If anti-K is of a very high titer, it is advisable to avoid using even the Red Blood Cells (because of the plasma around them) for transfusion purposes.

In Vitro Characteristics

The *in vitro* characteristics of anti-K are described in the following table.

The *In Vitro* Characteristics of Anti-K
• Is best detected by the antiglobulin test
• Occasionally reacts in saline
• May react at room temperature or lower
• Reactions not inhibited by enzyme treatment of red cells
• Some reports indicate reactivity is weakened in LISS/Coombs
• Does not typically show dosage

K as an Immunogen

K is considered to be a very good immunogen. Not only is the K antigen effective in causing people to produce anti-K, but most persons are K negative and are capable of being immunized if exposed to the antigen. In some donor centers within the United States, and even more commonly outside this country, it is a practice to type donor units for the K antigen and use the red cells selectively. About 9 percent of Caucasians are K positive compared to only 3 or 4 percent of the Black population.

Anti-K has been reported in the absence of exposure to red cells, but most of these patients suffered from an infection. Like the immune response to other natural antigens, the antibody in these cases was a saline agglutinin. In some of the cases the antibody disappeared as the patient recovered.

Some Interesting Facts

The Kell system is very interesting for a number of reasons. The genetics of the system appear to be somewhat like that of the Rh system; both are composed of a series of paired allelic genes occupying very closely linked loci. The amorphic gene K^o produces no Kell antigens. If K^o is inherited at both loci (K^o/K^o) no Kell antigens can be detected on the red cells. The phenotype is sometimes referred to as $Kell_{null}$.

In recent years several antibodies have been found that react with all cells tested except $Kell_{null}$ (K^o/K^o). This finding does not of itself establish that the antigen recognized by the antibody is part of the Kell system. Some of the antigens have been established to be part of the Kell system by statistical or family studies, but others have been assigned to the system only on a phenotypic level until further data confirm or exclude them.

Other rare Kell phenotypes were extensively studied when it was noted that weak Kell antigens were characteristic findings in some young males with X-linked chronic granulomatous disease (CGD). A dimension was added to this already fascinating study when it was discovered that adult males with a similar weakening of the Kell antigens (but without CGD) had greatly increased levels of creatine kinase in their plasma. Muscular abnormalities in one of these individuals led to an investigation which has revealed that similar problems are a common characteristic.

Other Antibodies of the Kell System

All other antibodies of the Kell system are extremely rare. Anti-k (anti-K2), the antibody which reacts with the antigen produced by the allele to K, is probably the most common. Even though k is a good immunogen, only 0.2 percent of the population are K/K and capable of producing the antibody. In a seven-year study in a major metropolitan transfusion service where 80,000 patients and donors were tested, only one anti-k was found. (Among antibodies to high-frequency antigens, anti-U, anti-Yt^a, anti-Kp^b, anti-Vel and others may be found more frequently than anti-k.)

Anti-Kp^a (anti-K3) is of little significance because it is rare and — even when present — is unlikely to be detected because only 2 percent of random donor bloods are Kp(a+).

7.5

Which are the significant antibodies of the Duffy system?

Clinically, the most important antibody of the Duffy system is anti-Fy^a. The clinical significance and *in vitro* characteristics of anti-Fy^a are described below. The relationship of the Duffy antigens to susceptibility to malaria is also discussed.

Clinical Significance

For transfusion candidates. Anti-Fy^a is among the more common antibodies found alone or in combination with other antibodies. Excluding anti-D, about 10 percent of clinically significant antibodies are anti-Fy^a. Anti-Fy^a has been reported frequently as a cause of extravascular transfusion reactions.

For obstetrical patients. If found in an obstetrical patient, anti-Fy^a should be regarded as a possible cause of hemolytic disease of the newborn and evaluated in the same way as other antibodies known to be IgG.

For donors. Plasma of donors with anti-Fy^a should be removed and the units used as Red Blood Cells.

In Vitro Characteristics

The *in vitro* characteristics of anti-Fy^a are described in the following table.

The *In Vitro* Characteristics of Anti-Fy^a
• Is best detected by the antiglobulin test
• May not react with ficin- or papain-treated red cells
• Does not typically exhibit dosage [Because of the high incidence of the amorph *Fy* in Blacks, it is difficult to know if an Fy(a+b−) cell is homozygous (Fy^a/Fy^a) or heterozygous (Fy^a/Fy).]

Fy^a as an Immunogen

Anti-Fy^a is produced as a result of red cell stimulation — there are no other known sources of the antigen. About 65 percent of Caucasians are Fy(a+) and 35 percent are Fy(a−); therefore, about one-third of all random persons are capable of producing anti-Fy^a if exposed to the antigen. In spite of the probability of exposure, anti-Fy^a is found in only a small percentage of transfused patients. The conclusion must be drawn that Fy^a is a poor immunogen. No attempt is made to match donors and non-immunized patients for the Fy^a antigen when transfusions are being given.

The incidence of the antigen is very different in Blacks: 65 percent are Fy(a–b–) and only 10 percent are Fy(a+). The incidence of the antibody is not increased in Blacks, however, because anti-Fy^a (or anti-Fy^b) is rarely produced by the Fy(a–b–) person.

Some Interesting Facts

It has been shown that the malarial parasite, *Plasmodium vivax*, does not invade red blood cells that are Fy(a–b–), regardless of the racial origin of the person. It would appear that the Duffy antigens or membrane structures closely related to them are the receptor sites for the invasion of this malarial parasite.

Other Antibodies of the Duffy System

Anti-Fy^b is a very rare antibody and when found it is often accompanied by other more common antibodies, such as anti-K or anti-c (hr′).

7.6

Which are the significant antibodies of the Kidd system?

The important antibodies of the Kidd system are anti-Jk^a and anti-Jk^b. Whereas anti-Jk^a is somewhat more common than anti-Jk^b, they both react *in vitro* and *in vivo* with similar characteristics. Unless otherwise stated the comments made here apply to either antibody.

Clinical Significance

For transfusion candidates. Although anti-Jk^a and anti-Jk^b are not as common as anti-K or anti-Fy^a, they are at least as significant for two reasons. They both characteristically fix complement; therefore, they can cause intravascular transfusion reactions. Secondly, they both tend to diminish in strength in the patient more rapidly than other antibodies. For this reason, they are often below a detectable level in the serum of a patient who is known to have been previously immunized. Under these conditions, antibody screening tests are negative and crossmatches may be serologically compatible even when tested with red blood cells carrying the corresponding antigen. A delayed transfusion reaction may result when such crossmatch-compatible, antigen-positive bloods are transfused. Delayed transfusion reactions are more often attributable to anti-Jk^a and anti-Jk^b than to any other antibody.

For obstetrical patients. Severe hemolytic disease of the newborn has been caused by anti-Jk^a and anti-Jk^b. Because these antibodies are found as frequently in Rh positive patients as in Rh negative patients, and because many Rh positive women are not screened for antibodies during pregnancy, the obstetrician may not be aware of the potential problem.

For donors. Anti-Jk^a is not likely to be found in a donor population because of its propensity to diminish in strength *in vivo*. If found, the plasma should be removed and the unit used as Red Blood Cells.

In Vitro Characteristics

The *in vitro* characteristics of anti-Jk^a and anti-Jk^b are summarized in the following table.

The *In Vitro* Characteristics of Anti-Jk^a and Anti-Jk^b
• Are detected by the antiglobulin test using polyspecific anti-human serum
• Often fix complement — may hemolyze test cells
• Reactivity frequently enhanced by using enzyme-treated cells
• Often show dosage

Jk^a and Jk^b as Immunogens

Persons who can produce anti-Jk^a number about the same as those who can produce anti-Jk^b, that is, about 25 percent. The relative rarity of the antibodies indicates that neither is an effective immunogen — Jk^b being even less immunogenic than Jk^a.

Antibody Levels

The most interesting aspect of the Kidd system is the failure of the antibody to remain at detectable levels following stimulation. The reason for this peculiarity is not entirely understood but may be related either to the subclass of antibody molecule or to the chemical nature of the antigen. This property makes the Kidd system particularly dangerous because the immunized patient may not be detected.

Other Antibodies of the Kidd System

Some persons, especially Orientals or Polynesians, are Jk(a–b–) and can produce anti-Jk3. This antibody reacts with all common phenotypes and fails to react with the rare Jk(a–b–) red cells. Serum containing anti-Jk3 often contains a separable anti-Jk^a or anti-Jk^b but anti-Jk3 is not simply a combination of the two antibodies in one serum.

7.7

Which are the significant antibodies of the MNSs system?

The two important antibodies of the MNSs system are anti-M and anti-S. The clinical significance and *in vitro* characteristics of each of these antibodies are discussed in this focus question.

Clinical Significance of Anti-M

For transfusion candidates. Each example of anti-M must be evaluated by its own characteristics to determine its clinical significance. Anti-M has been reported to cause transfusion reactions; however, many examples react only below 30°C and are not clinically significant.

For obstetrical patients. Anti-M has been the cause of hemolytic disease of the newborn in a few instances. Since it is now known that many examples of anti-M are totally IgG or have a large component of IgG, it is curious that it does not cause hemolytic disease of the newborn more frequently.

For donors. Unless reactive at 37°C and/or by the antiglobulin test, anti-M in a donor is of no significance. If the antibody reacts at 37°C, the plasma should be removed and the unit used as Red Blood Cells.

In Vitro Characteristics

The *in vitro* characteristics of anti-M are summarized in the following table.

The *In Vitro* Characteristics of Anti-M
• May react over a wide range of temperatures — some examples show typical cold agglutinin characteristics and others react at 37°C
• May be enhanced by the addition of albumin
• May be enhanced when low ionic solutions are added to the test system
• Very often shows some degree of dosage — often very pronounced
• Sometimes reactions are enhanced at pH 6.5
• Universally fails to react with enzyme-treated cells because the M antigen is removed from the cell surface by the action of proteolytic enzymes
• Many examples are primarily IgG. Their ability to agglutinate in saline or albumin is probably due to the density of the M antigen on red cells.

M as an Immunogen

About 22 percent of Caucasians are M negative and, if transfused with random blood, will often receive M positive blood. In spite of this the antibody is relatively rare because M is a poor immunogen. Most examples of anti-M are found in persons without known exposure to red blood cells.

Antigens of Low Frequency

Many antigens of low frequency are the products of genes whose loci are either closely linked to (or are a part of) the MN locus. Antibodies to some of these are quite common even though the corresponding antigen may be very rare. Among these are antibodies to the antigens of the Miltenberger subsystem collectively called anti-Mi.

Other Antibodies of the MNSs System

Anti-N is a very rare antibody. Some examples were found in hemodialysis patients regardless of whether the patient was N positive or N negative. It was believed that formaldehyde used to sterilize dialysis units was in some way related to the appearance of anti-N in these patients.

Clinical Significance of Anti-S

For transfusion candidates. Anti-S has caused hemolytic transfusion reactions.

For obstetrical patients. Hemolytic disease of the newborn has been caused by anti-S.

For donors. Donor bloods found to contain anti-S should be used as Red Blood Cells.

In Vitro Characteristics

The *in vitro* characteristics of anti-S are summarized in the following table.

The *In Vitro* Characteristics of Anti-S
• Best detected by the antiglobulin technique
• Occasional examples react with saline-suspended cells
• Reactivity not enhanced by enzymes — some enzymes will destroy the S antigen
• Can show dosage
• Producers of anti-S may not have had prior exposure to red cells

S as an Immunogen

Nearly one-half of Caucasians are S negative and, if transfused, could produce anti-S. The rarity of the antibody indicates that S is an inefficient immunogen.

Some Interesting Facts

Anti-s, which reacts with the antigen produced by the gene allelic to S, is not as common as anti-S. It has been the cause of hemolytic disease of the newborn and has the potential to cause transfusion reactions if incompatible blood is given.

About 2 percent of Blacks are S–s–. They can produce an antibody called anti-U which reacts with all red blood cells except those like the producer, that is, S–s–. Anti-U has caused transfusion reactions and hemolytic disease of the newborn.

7.8

Which are the significant antibodies of the P system?

Anti-P_1 is the most important antibody of the P system. Its clinical significance and *in vitro* characteristics are described below.

Clinical Significance

<u>For transfusion candidates.</u> Until recently anti-P_1 was probably the most commonly found cold alloagglutinin, but it is of very little clinical significance because the antibody rarely reacts above 30°C. The elimination of room temperature testing in antibody detection tests reduces the likelihood of finding anti-P_1. When detected in the serum of a patient, donors who are P_1 negative can be selected without great difficulty since about one in five donors is P_1 negative. It is highly unlikely that anti-P_1 will cause any difficulty in transfusion if the blood given is crossmatch-compatible. Anti-P_1 is less commonly found in Black patients because 90-95 percent of Blacks are P_1 positive compared to about 80 percent of Caucasians.

<u>For obstetrical patients.</u> Hemolytic disease of the newborn due to anti-P_1 has not been documented. The antibody is primarily IgM and cannot cross the placental barrier.

<u>For donors.</u> Donors whose sera contain anti-P_1 are of little concern.

In Vitro Characteristics

The *in vitro* characteristics of anti-P_1 are summarized in the following table.

The *In Vitro* Characteristics of Anti-P_1
• Usually reacts best below room temperature but may be detected at 20-25°C
• Reacts in saline but may be enhanced in albumin
• Agglutination is sometimes enhanced with enzyme-treated cells; enzymes do not destroy the P_1 antigen
• Strength of agglutination varies relative to the strength of the P_1 antigen
• Can be neutralized with ORTHO P_1 Blood Group Substance. Failure to observe reactions with P_1 positive cells after the addition of P_1 substance is positive identification of anti-P_1. Neutralization can also be an aid in identification when the antibody is in a mixture with other antibodies.

P₁ as an Immunogen

Exposure to P_1 positive red cells does not stimulate the production of anti-P_1; the antibody is found without regard to prior red blood cell exposure. If searched for with diligence, weak cold-reactive anti-P_1 may be found in nearly every P_1 negative person.

Chapter Eight:

In Vivo Reactions of Antigens and Antibodies

Objectives for Chapter Eight

Upon completion of this chapter you should be able to:

8.1
- **State the normal life span of red blood cells**

- **Discuss the following conditions which decrease the life span of red blood cells, causing hemolytic anemia:**
  - hereditary spherocytosis, hereditary elliptocytosis and hereditary stomatocytosis
  - glucose-6-phosphate dehydrogenase deficiency
  - sickle-cell anemia

8.2
- **Compare and contrast the major clinical effects of the following transfusion reactions:**
  - intravascular transfusion reactions
  - extravascular transfusion reactions
  - delayed transfusion reactions
  - febrile nonhemolytic reactions
  - anaphylactic reactions

8.3
- **Discuss the use of the following tests in diagnosing transfusion reactions:**
  - ABO testing
  - direct and indirect antiglobulin tests
  - plasma hemoglobin
  - plasma haptoglobin
  - hemoglobinuria
  - hemosiderinuria
  - bilirubin and urobilinogen

8.4
- **Describe the physiology of hemolytic disease of the newborn**

8.5
- **Discuss the following tests used to diagnose hemolytic disease of the newborn:**
  - blood grouping and typing
  - antibody screening and identification
  - maternal antibody titer
  - amniocentesis
  - direct antiglobulin test
  - cord hemoglobin
  - bilirubin determinations

- **Describe the role of Rh immune globulin in dramatically decreasing the incidence of hemolytic disease of the newborn**

8.1

What are the two major types of hemolytic anemia?

Anemia caused by excessive *in vivo* destruction of red blood cells (hemolysis) is called **hemolytic anemia**. A variety of inherited conditions may result in **congenital hemolytic anemia**. In addition, a number of acquired conditions may cause immunologically-mediated hemolytic anemia, usually referred to as **immune hemolytic anemia**. These two major types of hemolytic anemia are discussed below.

Congenital Hemolytic Anemia

Some of the more common inherited diseases that may cause hemolytic anemia are listed in Table 8.1A. As is seen in this table, these conditions can be divided into three groups: diseases affecting the red blood cell membrane, diseases affecting red blood cell metabolism (enzyme defects), and diseases affecting the structure of hemoglobin.

Table 8.1A Congenital conditions causing hemolytic anemia.

Diseases affecting the red blood cell membrane:
    Hereditary spherocytosis
    Hereditary elliptocytosis
    Hereditary stomatocytosis

Diseases affecting red blood cell metabolism:
    Glucose-6-phosphate dehydrogenase deficiency
    Pyruvate kinase deficiency

Diseases affecting the structure of hemoglobin:
    Sickle-cell anemia
    Thalassemia

Under normal conditions, the characteristic biconcave shape of the red blood cell membrane is maintained by a complex membrane skeleton consisting of a network of proteins on the internal side of the membrane adjacent to the hemoglobin. This skeletal network is believed to be attached to some of the proteins within the membrane. Genetic defects which alter the structure of these skeletal proteins result in abnormal red cell morphology. This is observed in the three congenital hemolytic anemias: **hereditary spherocytosis, hereditary elliptocytosis**, and **hereditary stomatocytosis**. **Sickle-cell anemia** is due to an abnormal hemoglobin, but also results in abnormal cell morphology.

The normal red blood cell life span is approximately 120 days. Senescent red blood cells lose their deformability and are trapped by the mesh-like structure of the spleen. The trapped cells are then phagocytized by splenic macrophages. Some constituents of the cell are reused. For example, the iron in hemoglobin is transported to the plasma iron storage pools to be used in various body functions, including hemoglobin synthesis. In hereditary spherocytosis, elliptocytosis and stomatocytosis, the abnormal red blood cell morphology causes premature sequestration and hemolysis in the spleen. Although the body may compensate by increasing the rate of red cell production, this shortened red blood cell life span usually results in some degree of anemia. In adults, the anemia is usually mild unless complicated by an **aplastic** crisis precipitated by infection. In severe disease, which is more common in the neonate, the plasma bilirubin level may become markedly elevated and an exchange transfusion may be required.

Several inherited enzyme defects cause alterations in red blood cell metabolism which may lead to congenital hemolytic anemia. For example, the enzyme **glucose-6-phosphate dehydrogenase (G6PD)** is known to exist in a number of variant forms that exhibit varying degrees of decreased activity of the enzyme. Decreased G6PD activity causes red cells to be more susceptible to oxidative denaturation. The red cells of newborns are normally more susceptible to oxidative denaturation than adult red cells. Certain forms of G6PD deficiency may exacerbate this condition, leading to severe **hyperbilirubinemia** in the newborn. An exchange blood transfusion may be required. Other variant forms of the enzyme may not produce any clinical signs or may produce hemolytic episodes only when the patient is exposed to the oxidant stress induced by certain drugs, such as the antimalarial drug primaquine. In these cases, the individual exhibits full recovery on withdrawal of the drug. Other variant forms of the enzyme appear to be responsible for hemolytic episodes that are not drug-induced. Deficiency of another enzyme, **pyruvate kinase (PK)**, alters the energy metabolism of red blood cells. Decreased energy production leads to cellular dehydration, altered cellular morphology, and a shortened red cell life span due to early destruction by the spleen.

Diseases in which the structure of the protein moiety of hemoglobin (globin) is altered are known as **hemoglobinopathies**. Probably the most common hemoglobinopathy is sickle-cell disease. The gene which controls the aberrant hemoglobin may be inherited either in the heterozygous (sickle-cell trait) or homozygous (sickle-cell disease) form. Hemoglobin is made of four polypeptide chains — two alpha chains and two beta chains. The substitution of valine for glutamate in the beta chains is responsible for the altered function of sickle-cell hemoglobin. Sickle-cell hemoglobin (Hb S) is capable of carrying molecular oxygen, but when it is deoxygenated, Hb S polymerizes into rigid structures that distort the red blood cells in the characteristic sickle shape. The sickled cells become trapped in the small blood vessels, leading to vaso-occlusion, microinfarction and organ damage. The damage to the red cell membrane leads to hemolysis of the cells which results in varying degrees of anemia (sickle-cell anemia). However, transfusions are given not so much to treat the anemia as to dilute the patient's sickle cells and decrease the resistance to blood flow caused by circulating abnormal cells.

It should be pointed out here that none of the congenital hemolytic anemias is associated with a positive direct antiglobulin test. The result of this test is often critical to the transfusion service when preparing blood for an exchange transfusion. In hemolytic disease of the newborn due to blood group incompatibility (immune hemolytic anemia), the direct antiglobulin test is usually positive and blood is selected according to the specificity of the antibody causing the disease. For an exchange transfusion of an infant suffering from congenital hemolytic anemia, selection of ABO-compatible and Rh-compatible blood is sufficient.

Immune Hemolytic Anemia

Immunologically-mediated hemolytic anemia may be caused by alloantibodies directed against foreign red cell antigens or by auto-antibodies directed against the patient's own red blood cells. As described in the earlier chapters of this book, alloantibodies are the result of a normal immune response following exposure to either antigenic substances resembling red blood cell antigens, as in the ABO system, or foreign red blood cells received through transfusion or fetal-maternal hemorrhage. While alloantibodies do not harm the patient's red cells, they can cause destruction of donor red cells carrying the corresponding antigen. In addition, maternal antibodies produced as a result of prior exposure to either donor or fetal red cells can cross the placenta and cause destruction of fetal red cells. The major purpose of the pretransfusion testing discussed throughout this book is to avoid conditions in which a patient with antibody is exposed to donor red cells carrying the corresponding antigen, and to prevent immunization to blood group antigens whenever possible.

Unlike alloantibodies, autoantibodies are the product of an abnormal immune response. They can destroy the patient's own red cells and the disease which results is called **autoimmune hemolytic anemia (AIHA)**. In autoimmune hemolytic anemia the source of stimulus of the autoantibodies is often unknown **(idiopathic)**. On the other hand, the causative agent is sometimes a drug or infectious agent and, in other cases, the production of autoantibodies may be secondary to another disease, such as **systemic lupus erythematosus (SLE)**, leukemia or **lymphoma**.

Autoantibodies directed against red cell antigens are either warm antibodies, whose optimal activity is about 37°C, or cold antibodies, whose optimal activity is below room temperature. In general, warm antibodies are IgG while cold antibodies are IgM. Warm autoantibodies, whether they be idiopathic or secondary, are often directed against antigens of the Rh system and cause little or no complement activation. Warm antibody-coated red blood cells are removed from the circulation by the spleen and, in severe cases, also by the liver. Depending on many factors which complicate autoimmune hemolytic anemia, hemolysis may be mild to severe and may be chronic or self-limited.

Autoimmune hemolytic anemia caused by cold agglutinins is called **cold agglutinin disease (CAD)** and the specificity of the antibody is usually anti-I. When cold antibodies are of high titer, the thermal range of activity increases and they may react up to 30°C. Under controlled laboratory conditions, cold autoagglutinins almost never react above 30°C. Cold antibodies can fix complement but because the thermal range of antibody activity is below body temperature, hemolysis is rare. In the extremities of the body the temperature is below 37°C and, when a person is exposed to a cold environment, peripheral temperatures may be much lower than the core temperature. Under these conditions people with cold agglutinin disease suffer hemolytic episodes. Cold agglutinin disease is relatively common following viral pneumonia. The symptoms may occur as late as a few weeks following apparent recovery from the pneumonia. During the disease the red cells lose their I antigen and extremely high titers of anti-I are produced. Upon recovery from the pneumonia, the newly formed red blood cells are I positive and a hemolytic crisis results. However, the hemolytic episode is self-limiting and transfusions are rarely required.

The **alpha-methyldopa** family of drugs sometimes causes the production of warm autoantibodies which frequently have Rh specificity. Even though the direct antiglobulin test may also be positive, hemolytic crises are very rare. After cessation of the drug therapy, the serological findings disappear slowly. When drugs other than alpha-methyldopa are involved in the etiology of autoimmune hemolytic anemia, the antibodies produced are not directed against red cell antigens but are directed either against the drug itself, which is tightly bound to the red cell, or against a drug complexed with protein. The drug-protein complex is only loosely adsorbed to the cells. The drug most often tightly bound to red cells is penicillin, and a drug-protein complex is typified by phenacetin. In both situations the red blood cell is considered an "innocent bystander." Conditions in which drug complexes are bound to the cell rarely result in hemolytic episodes, but the red cells have a positive direct antiglobulin test. A hemolytic crisis can be precipitated in the rare person who has anti-penicillin (IgG) when extremely large doses of penicillin are administered intravenously.

This focus question has provided an overview of hemolytic anemia — both congenital and immune — in order to place transfusion reactions and hemolytic disease of the newborn within the broader context of hemolytic anemias. These in vivo effects of alloantibodies are discussed in greater detail in the next focus question.

8.1 QUESTIONS

Anemia caused by excessive *in vivo* destruction of red blood cells is

called _____ .

hemolytic anemia

The normal biconcave structure of red blood cells is maintained by a complex network of proteins:

☐ internal to the cell membrane.

☐ external to the cell membrane.

internal to the cell membrane.

The normal red blood cell life span is approximately

_____ .

120 days

Senescent red blood cells are phagocytized by macrophages in the:

☐ kidney.

☐ spleen.

spleen.

The anemia of hereditary spherocytosis, elliptocytosis and stomatocytosis is due to:

☐ the shortened life span of the cells.

☐ the decreased oxygen-carrying capacity of the hemoglobin in the cells.

the shortened life span of the cells.

In these three conditions, the body usually attempts to compensate by

_____ .

increasing the rate of red cell production

A deficiency of the enzyme glucose-6-phosphate dehydrogenase causes red blood cells to:

☐ be more susceptible to oxidant stress.

☐ become elliptocytes.

be more susceptible to oxidant stress.

Hemoglobin S differs from normal hemoglobin:

☐ by the substitution of one amino acid in the beta chain.

☐ in the number of heme moieties.

by the substitution of one amino acid in the beta chain.

Which form of hemoglobin S polymerizes to form the structures which deform the red cells into a sickled shape?

☐ oxygenated

☐ deoxygenated

Match the following:

1 ____ sickle-cell trait   A homozygote

2 ____ sickle-cell disease   B heterozygote

Congenital hemolytic anemias

☐ are

☐ are not

associated with a positive direct antiglobulin test.

Match the following:

1 ____ autoantibodies   A normal immune response

2 ____ alloantibodies   B abnormal immune response

Antibodies that can destroy the patient's own red blood cells lead to

_____ hemolytic anemia.

Cold agglutinin disease is due to cold agglutinins which are:

☐ autoantibodies.

☐ alloantibodies.

The alpha-methyldopa family of drugs sometimes causes the production of warm autoantibodies which frequently have:

☐ Rh specificity.

☐ ABO specificity.

8.2

What are the major clinical effects of transfusion reactions?

The vast majority of transfusion reactions are the result of clerical errors and not the result of serological errors; for example, the blood specimen label did not properly reflect the patient from whom it was drawn, or blood prepared for one patient was administered to another. Such errors can have drastic consequences for the patient transfused with incompatible blood. Some reports indicate that as high as 40 to 50 percent of hemolytic transfusion reactions are fatal. This percentage will vary depending on how a hemolytic transfusion reaction is defined. Utmost care must be taken in performing tests in the blood bank, in recording test results, and in selecting and delivering blood for transfusions. Even more effort must be directed to finding better ways to identify patients and the blood specimens drawn from them.

Transfusion reactions can be divided into two types: intravascular and extravascular. In **intravascular transfusion reactions**, hemolysis takes place primarily in the bloodstream, and thus the clinical effect is immediate. Intravascular reactions are mediated by the activation of complement. Hemolysis occurs only if complement activation proceeds to completion. In contrast, **extravascular transfusion reactions** take place primarily in the spleen and/or occasionally in the liver. Clinical evidence of the reaction is somewhat slower and complement is not involved. In extravascular hemolysis, red blood cells are phagocytized by macrophages in the spleen or liver. These splenic or hepatic macrophages are part of a larger group of macrophages known collectively as the **reticuloendothelial system (RES)**, which is located in various organs of the body.

The prototype of an intravascular transfusion reaction is one resulting from the transfusion of ABO-incompatible blood. Anti-A and anti-B are IgM and fix complement, leading to brisk intravascular hemolysis. The antibody binding, complement activation and cell lysis occurring in intravascular hemolysis are illustrated in Figure 8.2A.

The clinical manifestations of an intravascular transfusion reaction usually appear within minutes after the transfusion is started. Typically, the patient complains of a burning sensation at the site of infusion and the pain may spread rapidly to the lower back and to the area of the sternum. Flushing, fever, chills, difficulty in breathing, and a sudden drop in blood pressure may also occur. In severe cases, the patient's condition may progress rapidly to shock, disseminated intravascular coagulation and renal failure.

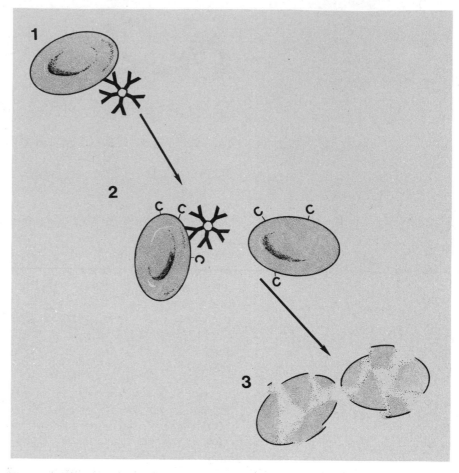

Figure 8.2A Illustration of intravascular hemolysis. (1) Binding of IgM antibodies to red blood cells. (2) Complement activation. (3) Red cell lysis.

In contrast to intravascular transfusion reactions, extravascular transfusion reactions usually involve antibodies other than anti-A and/or anti-B, e.g., antibodies of the Rh, Kell or Duffy system. The antibodies involved are usually IgG and they rarely fix complement. The coating of donor red blood cells with IgG antibodies and their subsequent phagocytosis by reticuloendothelial cells are illustrated in Figure 8.2B.

In general, extravascular transfusion reactions are less severe than intravascular transfusion reactions. Since the destruction of senescent red blood cells is an ongoing function of the spleen, the threshold of normal destruction must be surpassed before increased destruction due to a transfusion reaction results in clinical symptoms. For this reason, a delay ranging from minutes to hours may occur between the initiation of the transfusion and the clinical manifestations of an extravascular reaction. The length of this delay will depend upon a number of factors, including the patient's antibody titer, the type of antibody, and the general physical condition of the patient. Needless to say, a severely debilitated patient will suffer more than a "healthier" patient. The clinical manifestations of extravascular transfusion reactions are often limited to fever, chills and back pain. However, unless recognized and properly treated, renal complications can be one of the unfortunate sequelae of red cell destruction.

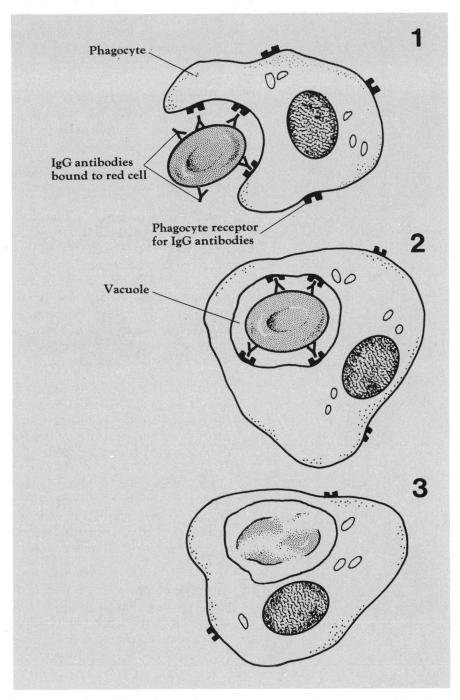

Figure 8.2B Illustration of extravascular hemolysis. (1) IgG antibodies bound to the red cell interact with receptors on the membrane of a phagocytic cell. (2) Phagocyte engulfs the antibody-coated red blood cell, incorporating it into an intracellular vacuole. (3) Lysis of the red cell occurs within the intracellular vacuole of the phagocyte.

Delayed transfusion reactions can be difficult to diagnose. They occur when a patient previously sensitized to red blood cell antigens has undetectable antibodies at the time of transfusion. Under these conditions, incompatible blood will not be recognized as such in the crossmatch procedure but, since the patient is immunized,* antibodies may be rapidly restimulated (anamnestic response). The clinical symptoms of the transfusion reaction may not appear until two to three days or as long as two to three weeks after the transfusion. Delayed transfusion reactions are always extravascular; they may be mild to moderately severe, but in most cases therapy is not required. Occasionally a delayed transfusion reaction is severe and requires treatment; at least one death has been reported, probably because the reaction was unrecognized in the early stages.

In addition to intravascular and extravascular transfusion reactions, two other types of transfusion reactions should be mentioned briefly.

Febrile nonhemolytic reactions are due to the presence of antibodies to white blood cell or platelet antigens. They are observed only in patients who have been multiply transfused or have had multiple pregnancies. Febrile nonhemolytic reactions usually occur within minutes of the time the transfusion is started. Symptoms include fever, chills and malaise, and the reaction may resemble the early stages of an acute hemolytic transfusion reaction. Febrile nonhemolytic reactions are common and they are important because they must be distinguished from acute life-threatening hemolytic transfusion reactions. The fever usually responds to **antipyretic** therapy.

Anaphylactic reactions may occur in very rare patients who are IgA-deficient and have developed anti-IgA antibodies. In such patients the reaction occurs in response to the infusion of IgA — a normal plasma protein present in donor blood. Anaphylactic reactions are dramatic and occur after the infusion of only a few milliliters of blood or plasma. Gastrointestinal upset may be the first symptom to appear, but a sudden drop in blood pressure usually occurs within minutes. Immediate recognition and treatment are required or death can result. When a patient has had an anaphylactic transfusion reaction, subsequent transfusions must be limited to red cells that have been thoroughly washed to remove any IgA. No plasma or plasma products can be tolerated.

At the first signs of any transfusion reaction, the transfusion should be stopped and the attention of a physician sought immediately. A sample of the patient's blood, as well as the bag containing the unused blood, should be sent to the transfusion laboratory in order to determine whether incompatibility is the cause of the reaction.

*The term **sensibilized** is sometimes applied to the state of immunization in which no antibodies can be detected.

8.2 QUESTIONS

Most transfusion reactions result from:

☐ serological errors.

☐ clerical errors.

State whether each of the following is more characteristic of intravascular or extravascular transfusion reactions:

occurs primarily in the spleen and/or occasionally in the liver

_____

requires complete complement activation

_____

clinical effects are seen immediately

_____

red blood cells are phagocytized by macrophages in the spleen or liver

_____

The reticuloendothelial system consists of

☐ reticulocytes

☐ macrophages

located in various organs of the body.

Transfusion of ABO-incompatible blood leads to:

☐ intravascular hemolysis.

☐ extravascular hemolysis.

Anti-A and anti-B which fix complement are:

☐ IgM

☐ IgG

The clinical manifestations of an intravascular transfusion reaction usually appear within:

☐ minutes.

☐ hours.

clerical errors.

extravascular

intravascular

intravascular

extravascular

macrophages

intravascular hemolysis.

IgM

minutes.

In an acute intravascular transfusion reaction the patient typically complains of a burning sensation at _____ .

The pain may spread rapidly to _____

_____ .

The patient typically has:

☐ fever, chills, flushing and difficulty in breathing.

☐ no difficulty in breathing and is pale.

In an acute transfusion reaction, blood pressure may often:

☐ fall.

☐ rise.

Rh, Kell or Duffy antibodies are most likely to cause:

☐ intravascular transfusion reactions.

☐ extravascular transfusion reactions.

Which type of transfusion reaction is usually more severe?

☐ intravascular transfusion reactions

☐ extravascular transfusion reactions

If an extravascular transfusion reaction is not recognized and treated, _____ complications can be one of the unfortunate sequelae of red cell destruction.

Delayed transfusion reactions typically occur when the patient has been sensitized to red cell antigens and has antibodies that are

☐ detectable

☐ undetectable

at the time of transfusion.

The clinical symptoms of a delayed transfusion reaction usually occur

☐ hours to days

☐ days to weeks

after the transfusion.

Delayed transfusion reactions are always:

☐ intravascular.

☐ extravascular.

In a delayed transfusion reaction, therapy usually:

☐ is required.

☐ is not required.

Febrile nonhemolytic reactions are due to antibodies to:

☐ white blood cell and platelet antigens.

☐ tissue macrophage antigens.

A febrile nonhemolytic reaction is most likely to cause confusion by appearing as the early stages of:

☐ an acute hemolytic transfusion reaction.

☐ a delayed transfusion reaction.

Anaphylactic reactions typically occur in rare patients who have:

☐ anti-IgM.

☐ anti-IgA.

Anaphylactic reactions

☐ do

☐ do not

require therapy.

by thoroughly washing red cells to remove all IgA

Once recognized, how can anaphylactic reactions be avoided?

_____

_____

What should be done when the symptoms of a transfusion reaction are recognized?

_____

_____

_____

_____

_____

_____

_____

_____

The transfusion should be stopped immediately and a physician should be called. The bag containing the unused blood and a sample of the patient's blood should be sent to the laboratory to see whether incompatibility is the cause of the reaction.

8.3

What tests are used to diagnose transfusion reactions?

When a transfusion reaction is suspected, a variety of blood bank and clinical laboratory tests may be performed. Prior to any laboratory testing, the most important task is to examine all records to determine if the patient who received the blood is the patient for whom the blood was crossmatched, and if the unit of blood given to the patient bears the same identification number as that recorded from the segments used for the crossmatch. The precise protocol for investigating a transfusion reaction can be found elsewhere. The intention here is to describe reasons for performing the tests. The particular tests used in a blood bank and clinical laboratory will vary, but certain tests are standard. Those that are commonly used are described below.

ABO Testing

Because the severity of a transfusion reaction due to incompatibility in the ABO system is greater than that in other blood group systems, prompt treatment is critical to prevent shock and resultant renal damage. For this reason, the first tests run are those to check ABO grouping. Both pretransfusion and posttransfusion specimens of the patient should be tested, as well as red blood cells from the segments used in the original crossmatch and red blood cells from the blood bag.

Direct and Indirect Antiglobulin Tests

At the time of a transfusion reaction, the direct antiglobulin test may or may not be positive, depending upon the type of antibody involved in the reaction and the degree of cell lysis at the time the specimen is drawn. A positive direct antiglobulin test usually indicates the presence of recipient antibodies on the surface of donor red blood cells, but occasionally the positive direct antiglobulin test is due to infusion of many packs of ABO-incompatible platelets. In the latter situation, red cell destruction rarely occurs but the positive direct antiglobulin test may cause confusion in interpreting other evidence of a hemolytic transfusion reaction.

A positive antibody screening test (indirect antiglobulin test) indicates the presence of free antibodies in the patient's serum. The antibody screening test will be negative only if all the antibodies are bound to red blood cells. This may be the situation immediately following the transfusion; however, the antibody will reappear in the serum, usually within a few hours and almost certainly within a few days.

If there is evidence of antibody either free in the patient's serum or attached to the donor red blood cells (or both), identification tests should be performed in order to determine the exact cause of the incompatibility. It is always advisable to prepare an eluate using posttransfusion blood drawn from the patient (which contains donor cells also) because the offending antibody is most likely to be found in the eluate. As a final confirmation, segments from the units given should be tested for the antigen or antigens corresponding to the antibodies identified in the patient's serum or in the eluate.

Plasma Hemoglobin

In an intravascular transfusion reaction, hemoglobin is released directly into the bloodstream. Hemoglobin in the plasma binds to a protein called **haptoglobin** which transports the hemoglobin to the reticuloendothelial system where it is catabolized. In intravascular hemolysis the binding capacity of haptoglobin is rapidly saturated. As a result, the level of free plasma hemoglobin rises. The destruction of even a few milliliters of red blood cells will raise the plasma hemoglobin level sufficiently to be visible with the naked eye. As shown in Figure 8.3A, an increase in the plasma hemoglobin level is characteristic of intravascular hemolysis. Except in circumstances of gross red blood cell destruction, plasma hemoglobin levels are normal in extravascular hemolysis.

Plasma Haptoglobin

As the plasma haptoglobin becomes saturated with hemoglobin, the complex is taken up by the reticuloendothelial system and the plasma haptoglobin level decreases rapidly. Like the increase in plasma hemoglobin, the decrease in plasma haptoglobin is usually seen in intravascular hemolysis. It must be remembered that there are many circumstances in which haptoglobin is low, and a low posttransfusion haptoglobin is meaningful only when compared with the pretransfusion value. Even the administration of large quantities of bank blood near outdate will drastically reduce the haptoglobin level in a recipient.

Hemoglobinuria and Hemosiderinuria

Free hemoglobin in the plasma is filtered by the kidneys and excreted in the urine. Thus, hemoglobinuria occurs following intravascular hemolysis. The renal involvement following a transfusion reaction is due to hypotension in which the blood flow to the kidneys is severely restricted. Although free hemoglobin is found in the kidney tubules, it is not the cause of the **ischemia** because hemoglobin itself is not toxic. When hemolysis is chronic, as is common in autoimmune hemolytic anemia, the heme iron deposited in renal cells is stored in the form of a pigment called **hemosiderin**. Hemosiderin in the urine indicates chronic red blood cell destruction. Hemosiderin may also be deposited in the liver, heart and endocrine glands, eventually causing failure of their functions.

Bilirubin and Urobilinogen

Bilirubin, the breakdown product of the heme portion of hemoglobin, is released into the circulation where it binds to albumin and is carried to the liver. In the liver, bilirubin is conjugated with sugar residues to make it more soluble and more readily excreted in the bile. This conjugation of bilirubin with glucuronates is an enzymatic reaction involving glucuronyltransferase.* In *both* intravascular and

---

*This enzyme is not developed in newborns. The lack of glucuronyltransferase accounts for the inability of the newborn to excrete bilirubin and the resultant dangers of hyperbilirubinemia and kernicterus.

extravascular hemolysis, the plasma level of unconjugated bilirubin is elevated as shown in Figure 8.3A. The presence of bilirubin in plasma is rarely observed in less than six hours. For this reason, tests for plasma bilirubin need not be performed on posttransfusion specimens drawn immediately after the reaction, but another specimen should be drawn at six to eight hours for this test. In hyperbilirubinemia, bilirubin pigments are deposited in the body tissues, causing clinical jaundice. Conjugated bilirubin excreted in the bile is converted by intestinal bacteria to **urobilinogen**, which is then excreted in the feces. Thus, stool urobilinogen levels may be elevated in both intravascular and extravascular hemolysis.

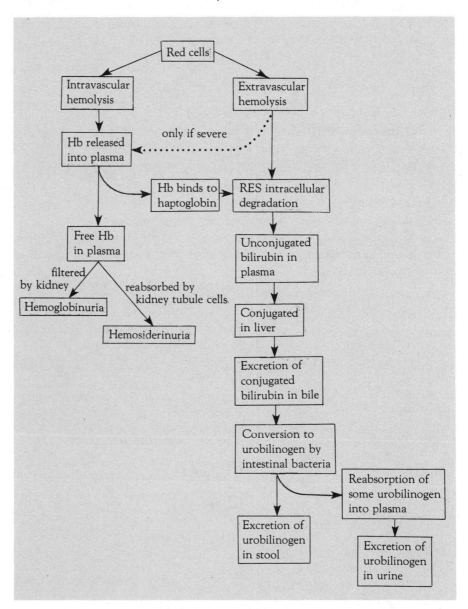

Figure 8.3A The fate of hemoglobin and its degradation products in intravascular and extravascular hemolysis. Abbreviations: Hb–hemoglobin; RES–reticuloendothelial system.

8.3 QUESTIONS

When a transfusion reaction is suspected, prior to any laboratory testing, it is important to

_____

_____

_____

_____ .

Transfusion reactions are likely to be most severe in:

☐ Rh incompatibility.

☐ ABO incompatibility.

When an ABO-incompatible transfusion reaction is suspected, it is important to test

☐ only posttransfusion

☐ both pretransfusion and posttransfusion

specimens of the patient's blood.

A positive direct antiglobulin test at the time of a transfusion reaction usually indicates the presence of

☐ donor

☐ recipient

antibodies on the surface of

☐ donor

☐ recipient

red blood cells.

A positive indirect antiglobulin test indicates the presence of

_____ antibodies in the patient's serum.

Immediately after an acute transfusion reaction, the antibody screening test (indirect antiglobulin test) may be negative because

all the antibodies are bound to donor red cells

_____

_____ .

Once an antibody (either free or attached to the donor red cells) has been detected in a transfusion reaction, identification tests:

should be performed.

☐ should be performed.

☐ are not of any value.

Hemoglobin released from red cells in an intravascular transfusion

haptoglobin

reaction binds to a serum protein called _____ ,
which transports the hemoglobin to the reticuloendothelial system where it is catabolized.

The level of free hemoglobin in the plasma usually rises in:

intravascular hemolysis.

☐ intravascular hemolysis.

☐ extravascular hemolysis.

☐ both

In intravascular hemolysis, plasma haptoglobin levels usually:

☐ increase.

decrease.

☐ decrease.

Free hemoglobin in the plasma is excreted by the:

☐ liver.

☐ spleen.

kidneys.

☐ kidneys.

The pigment resulting from the deposition of iron in renal cells due to

hemosiderin

chronic hemolysis is called _____ .

hypotension and reduced renal blood flow.

bilirubin

bilirubin

both

liver.

glucuronyltransferase

Following a transfusion reaction, renal complications are due to:

☐ hypotension and reduced renal blood flow.

☐ the toxic effects of hemoglobin on renal tubular cells.

The breakdown product of the heme portion of hemoglobin is called

_____.

Jaundice is caused by the deposition of

☐ hemosiderin

☐ bilirubin

in body tissues.

The plasma level of unconjugated bilirubin is elevated in:

☐ intravascular hemolysis.

☐ extravascular hemolysis.

☐ both

Normally, bilirubin is conjugated and excreted by the:

☐ liver.

☐ spleen.

☐ kidneys.

Newborns are more prone to hyperbilirubinemia because they lack

the enzyme _____,
which is required to conjugate bilirubin before it is excreted.

8.4

What are the physiologic characteristics of hemolytic disease of the newborn?

In many ways, hemolytic disease of the newborn (**HDN**) is a transfusion reaction in which antibodies produced by the mother cause the destruction of fetal red blood cells. The effect of maternal antibodies on fetal red cells differs, however, from a transfusion reaction in an adult because of the unique relationship between fetal and maternal circulations.

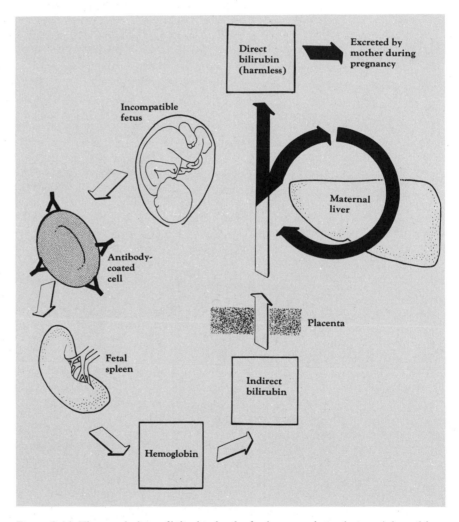

Figure 8.4A The metabolism of bilirubin by the fetal-maternal circulation. Adapted from *Blood Group Antigens & Antibodies as Applied to Hemolytic Disease of the Newborn*, Ortho Diagnostic Systems, 1968.

In utero the reticuloendothelial system of the fetus destroys the fetal red cells sensitized with maternal antibody, and the waste products are transported via the placenta to the mother's circulation and excreted. To compensate for the red cell destruction, the fetal bone marrow produces more red blood cells; in severe cases, the liver may be diverted to **extramedullary hemopoiesis** in an attempt to compensate. Decreased normal liver function may cause **hypoproteinemia** and severe tissue **edema.** In addition, the anemia of the fetus places an extra strain on the fetal circulatory system, and this may lead to congestive heart failure. In the most severe cases, the fetus may die *in utero.* **Hydrops fetalis** is the term used to describe the condition of a fetus with severe anemia, congestive heart failure, an enlarged liver and pronounced edema. Hydropic infants are usually stillborn but if alive are rarely, if ever, saved. Fortunately, the majority of babies with hemolytic disease of the newborn are not as severely affected as described above, but **kernicterus** may develop within a few hours of birth if the plasma bilirubin levels become too high. For this reason, hemolytic disease of the newborn must be diagnosed and treated before irreversible brain damage occurs.

8.4 QUESTIONS

In hemolytic disease of the newborn

maternal

☐ fetal

☐ maternal

antibodies sensitize the fetal red blood cells.

These sensitized red blood cells are then destroyed by the

fetal

☐ fetal

☐ maternal

reticuloendothelial system.

The products of red cell destruction are then transported via the

placenta

_____ to the mother's circulation and excreted.

In hemolytic disease of the newborn, the fetal bone marrow produces

more

☐ more

☐ fewer

red blood cells.

Extramedullary hemopoiesis means that organs other than bone

red blood cells

marrow are diverted to producing _____ .

The resulting decrease in normal liver function causes hypo-proteinemia and severe tissue:

☐ dehydration.

edema.

☐ edema.

The extra strain placed on the fetal circulation may cause:

congestive heart failure.

☐ congestive heart failure.

☐ increased cardiac output.

can	Severe hemolytic disease of the newborn
	☐ can
	☐ cannot
	cause death *in utero*.
	When an infant with hemolytic disease is born with severe anemia, congestive heart failure, an enlarged liver and pronounced edema, the
hydrops fetalis	condition is called _____ .
	These infants
	☐ sometimes
rarely, if ever,	☐ rarely, if ever,
	survive.
	Most babies with hemolytic disease of the newborn
	☐ are
are not	☐ are not
	born with hydrops fetalis.
	It is particularly important to diagnose and treat hemolytic disease of the newborn because severely elevated bilirubin levels can cause
kernicterus	_____ ,
	which results in irreversible damage to the brain.

8.5

What tests are used to diagnose hemolytic disease of the newborn?

Testing for evidence of hemolytic disease of the newborn can be divided into two stages: (1) during pregnancy to determine fetal risk, and (2) after birth to diagnose hemolytic disease of the newborn. These two stages of testing are described below.

Testing During Pregnancy

All pregnant women should be tested to determine whether they are Rh positive or Rh negative. While Rh blood group incompatibility caused most cases of hemolytic disease of the newborn in the past, the incidence of the disease has been reduced dramatically due to the use of Rh immune globulin. However, hemolytic disease of the newborn caused by other blood group incompatibilities is no less common than in the past, and is as likely to be found in Rh positive as in Rh negative women. For this reason, all pregnant women should be screened for antibodies at least once during pregnancy, and Rh negative women should be screened at least twice. The first test on an Rh negative woman should be performed early in pregnancy and the second at about 28 weeks. When Rh immune globulin is to be administered as antepartum prophylaxis at 28 weeks, the blood sample for antibody screening should be drawn prior to the injection, although it need not be tested until later. Since the vast majority of women are not immunized, it is not necessary to wait for the results of screening tests to identify the rare Rh negative woman who does not need Rh immune globulin. Rh immune globulin will do no harm to a woman who is already immunized.

Some women of childbearing age have anti-D in their sera in spite of efforts to eradicate immunization. Titration of the anti-D or other significant antibodies in the mother's blood is performed to assess the risk of disease in the infant. If the maternal antibody titer is below a critical level, the risk is minimal and amniocentesis should not be performed. Each laboratory must establish its own critical antibody titer based on the particular test procedure used. The critical titer can be set as that titer below which clinically serious hemolytic disease of the newborn has not occurred in the patient population served by that laboratory. When the maternal antibody titer rises above the established level (usually a titer of 16 or 32), amniocentesis is indicated to more accurately assess the condition of the fetus. Amniocentesis, as illustrated in Figure 8.5A, is a surgical procedure in which a sample of amnionic fluid is withdrawn for laboratory analysis. The procedure should be performed using ultrasound imaging of the fetus in order to avoid puncturing the placenta or injuring the fetus with the sampling needle.

Some fetal red blood cells may enter the maternal circulation during amniocentesis no matter how carefully the procedure is performed, increasing the risk of additional antibody production. For this reason, amniocentesis should not be performed without careful consideration of the serological status of the patient.

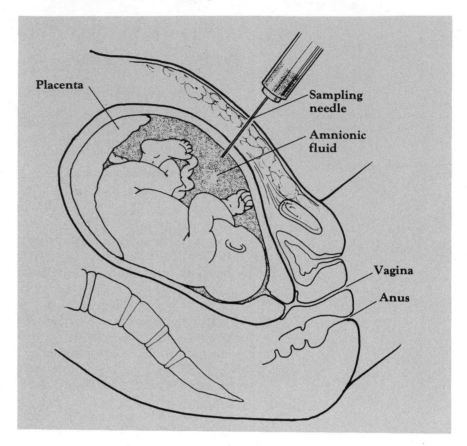

Figure 8.5A Illustration of amniocentesis.

Excessive hemolysis of fetal red blood cells will result in an increased level of hemoglobin breakdown products in the amnionic fluid. Bilirubin, the principal hemoglobin breakdown product, enters the amnionic fluid primarily by **transudation** through the blood vessels of the umbilical cord. In addition, some bilirubin is regurgitated from the fetal gastrointestinal tract into the amnionic fluid, and a small amount is excreted by the fetal kidneys. The bilirubin level in amnionic fluid samples is measured by scanning spectrophotometric analysis.

Three levels of bilirubin in amnionic fluid have been defined. The same level varies in significance depending on the gestational age of the fetus as illustrated in the graph in Figure 8.5B. A high bilirubin level indicates a significant degree of hemolysis and fetal anemia. If it is believed that the fetus will not survive to term, intrauterine blood transfusions are given to the fetus to alleviate the anemia. A moderate bilirubin level indicates that the fetus is at significant risk of hemolytic disease of the newborn, and early delivery and immediate exchange transfusion are usually sufficient to save these babies.

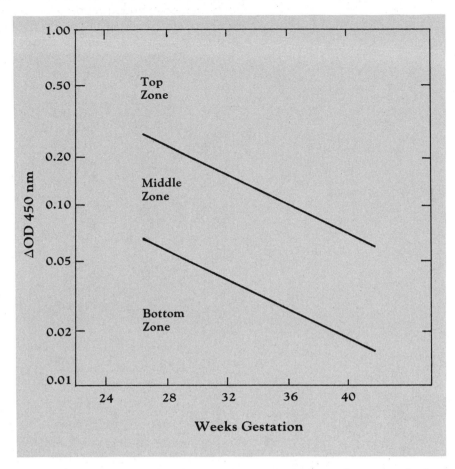

Figure 8.5B When the results of spectrophotometric analyses of amnionic fluid are plotted in this graph, the severity of the disease can be evaluated. Results falling in the top zone indicate a severely affected baby who may require intrauterine transfusions or immediate delivery, depending on the gestational age and maturity of the infant. Results falling in the bottom zone indicate mildly affected infants, and results falling in the middle zone should be considered cautiously.

In contrast to Rh incompatibility, there are no tests to predict hemolytic disease due to ABO incompatibility, which often occurs in the first-born and may or may not occur in subsequent pregnancies. The diagnosis of hemolytic disease due to ABO incompatibility is made after delivery, often on the basis of exclusion of all other possible explanations for the child's condition. Although the serological picture in ABO incompatibility is not as clear-cut as in hemolytic disease due to Rh incompatibility, there are very definite signs that may be used as diagnostic aids by the pediatrician.

Testing After Birth
When prenatal investigation of the maternal serum has disclosed the presence of an atypical blood group antibody capable of causing hemolytic disease, clinical examination of the infant is directed toward determining whether the antibody has affected the child, the severity of the disease, and the necessity for treatment. If results of antibody

screening tests on the prenatal patient were negative, or if such tests were not performed, the problem becomes one of differentiating jaundice and anemia due to blood group incompatibility from that due to other causes. Some of these other causes are listed in Table 8.5C and include **physiological jaundice** of the newborn and the congenital hemolytic anemias described at the beginning of this chapter.

Table 8.5C Causes of neonatal jaundice other than hemolytic disease due to blood group incompatibility.

Physiologic	Hyperbilirubinemia of premature infants
	Hereditary spherocytosis
	Congenital hemolytic anemia
Metabolic	Maternal diabetes
	Galactosemia
	G6PD deficiency
	Pyruvate kinase deficiency
Infections	Congenital syphilis
	Hepatitis
	Rubella
	Cytomegalic inclusion disease
Drugs	Overdose of vitamin K
	Naphthalene

The Direct Antiglobulin Test

A direct antiglobulin test (direct Coombs test) on blood of the infant provides valuable evidence to support or negate a diagnosis of hemolytic disease of the newborn due to blood group incompatibility. Ideally, a direct antiglobulin test should be performed on the cord blood of all newborns. This could save hours of delay in the recognition of hemolytic disease of the newborn, especially in those infants whose mothers have received no prenatal care. Unless the mother is known to be immunized, such tests need not be performed on an emergency basis but could be part of the daily procedures of the laboratory. If direct antiglobulin testing is not considered feasible for all babies, one might substitute routine collection and refrigerated storage of cord blood. If there are signs of trouble, then cord blood is available for investigation. In certain situations, such as hemolytic disease due to ABO incompatibility, a positive direct antiglobulin test is much more likely on cord blood than on a sample drawn after clinical signs develop. The cord specimen should be collected either with a needle and syringe, or by simple flow from the cut end of the cord without undue stripping. Careful collection prevents contamination with Wharton's jelly or tissue fluids that might interfere with testing.

The finding of a positive direct antiglobulin test confirms that the child's red blood cells have absorbed maternal antibody. When an antibody has been detected and identified in the mother's serum during pregnancy, it is usually assumed that this is the antibody attached to the infant's red cells. If desired, the antibody specificity may be confirmed by elution studies. Eluates can be especially helpful in

ABO hemolytic disease of the newborn. Elution of antibody from the child's red blood cells (anti-A, for instance, from the red blood cells of a group A baby) is strong evidence for a diagnosis of ABO hemolytic disease.

In addition to the direct antiglobulin test, a simple procedure which has been found invaluable in confirming ABO hemolytic disease is the test of the cord serum for antibody that is antagonistic to the child's red blood cells. Finding free circulating anti-A in the serum of a group A baby suggests that the tissues and red blood cells are saturated with antibody and can absorb no more.

When no prenatal testing has been done, or testing was negative and the newborn shows a positive direct antiglobulin test, one should obtain blood from the mother for grouping, typing and antibody identification. A blood sample from the father, if group-compatible with the mother, may aid in the identification of an antibody to a low-incidence antigen. If the mother's blood is not available, tests of the cord serum and an eluate made from the cord cells will often establish the identity of the antibody responsible for the child's condition. The eluate can also be used for crossmatching when maternal serum cannot be obtained. Cord serum and eluates should be tested in the same way as maternal serum.

The direct antiglobulin test may be negative on the red blood cells of a baby whose mother is known to have an antibody. If the test was properly performed, the red blood cells have not absorbed the maternal antibody and the child would be expected to be healthy. Either the antibody did not pass the placental barrier or the fetal red blood cells lack the antigen against which the antibody is directed.

A diseased baby who has received intrauterine transfusions may have a negative direct antiglobulin test and may also appear to be Rh negative at delivery; however, this does not mean that jaundice will not develop. The child must be watched carefully and its condition should be monitored by hemoglobin and bilirubin determinations.

Once it is established that a baby is suffering from hemolytic disease, the identity of the maternal antibody becomes important in the selection of blood for a possible exchange transfusion, since the blood to be used should be compatible with the antibody causing the child's condition. Knowledge of the identity of the antibody allows one to test the cells of prospective donors to determine that they lack the corresponding antigen, rather than relying solely on the crossmatch.

The strength of reaction of a positive direct antiglobulin test does not indicate the severity of the disease process. Hemoglobin and indirect bilirubin levels are better measures of the extent of red blood cell destruction and elimination.

Cord Hemoglobin

The degree of anemia depends on the ability of the infant to produce new red blood cells to replace those destroyed. If increased **erythropoiesis** has allowed the child to keep pace with red blood cell destruction, hemoglobin levels may be relatively normal despite some degree of jaundice. Cord hemoglobin values below 14 g/dL are considered abnormal and are suggestive of a hemolytic process. Severely affected infants may have cord hemoglobin levels as low as 3 or 4 g/dL. In hemolytic disease due to ABO incompatibility, hemoglobin values are often close to normal since anemia is not usually a diagnostic symptom of the disease.

Bilirubin Determinations

Peak levels of bilirubin are usually attained by the third day of life in full-term babies and may reach 40 to 50 mg/dL in untreated cases of hemolytic disease. Levels in normal full-term infants seldom exceed 13 mg/dL at 48 hours of age, but premature babies with physiological jaundice may have serum bilirubins as high as 30 mg/dL. By the third or fourth day, the liver of the full-term infant produces sufficient glucuronyltransferase to convert bilirubin to its excretable form — bilirubin diglucuronide — and the bilirubin levels in serum are reduced. While the risk of kernicterus seems to be greatest in infants with serum bilirubin in excess of 20 mg/dL, low motor and/or mental scores may result from neonatal hyperbilirubinemia of 16 to 19 mg/dL.

Because of the virtual eradication of Rh hemolytic disease of the newborn, exchange transfusions are usually performed only in hospitals equipped for special prenatal and perinatal care. Selection of blood for exchange transfusion is discussed in many other texts.

8.5 QUESTIONS

Rh testing should be done on

- ☐ all

- ☐ only high risk

pregnant women.

all

The incidence of hemolytic disease of the newborn has been greatly

reduced by the use of _____ .

Rh immune globulin

Which group of women should be tested more than once during their pregnancy?

- ☐ Rh positive

- ☐ Rh negative

Rh negative

The first test should be performed early in the pregnancy and the second test on an Rh negative woman should be performed at

_____ weeks.

28

When Rh immune globulin is being administered as antepartum prophylaxis, the blood sample for antibody screening should be drawn

- ☐ before

- ☐ after

before

administration of Rh immune globulin; however, the antibody screening test

- ☐ must

- ☐ need not

need not

be done before the injection.

when the mother's antibody titer is greater than 16 to 32

When should amniocentesis be used to assess the condition of the fetus?

_____

_____

can

Fetal red blood cells

☐ can

☐ cannot

enter the maternal circulation during amniocentesis.

Bilirubin levels in amnionic fluid are

increased

☐ increased

☐ decreased

in hemolytic disease of the newborn.

When hemolytic disease of the newborn is so severe that it is believed the fetus will not survive to term, what therapy is used to alleviate the fetal anemia?

intrauterine blood transfusions

_____

_____

The diagnosis of hemolytic disease of the newborn due to ABO incompatibility is made:

☐ during pregnancy.

at birth.

☐ at birth.

In hemolytic disease of the newborn, a positive direct antiglobulin test is more likely using the infant's:

cord blood.

☐ cord blood.

☐ blood drawn after clinical signs of the disease develop.

In confirming ABO hemolytic disease, the finding of free antibodies in the cord serum which are antagonistic to the child's red blood cells suggests that the child's tissues and red cells

☐ are

☐ are not

saturated with antibody.

Once hemolytic disease of the newborn is established, the identity of the maternal antibody:

☐ is important.

☐ is not important.

This is because of the possibility that the child may require a(n)

_____ .

Cord hemoglobin levels below

☐ 18 g/dL

☐ 14 g/dL

are considered abnormal and suggest a hemolytic process.

In normal full-term babies, bilirubin levels usually peak by the

_____ day of life.

In a normal full-term baby, bilirubin levels rarely exceed

☐ 23 mg/dL

☐ 13 mg/dL

at 48 hours.

The risk of kernicterus is greatest in infants with serum bilirubin in

excess of _____ mg/dL.

are

is important.

exchange transfusion.

14 g/dL

third

13 mg/dL

20

Glossary

agglutination . . . . clumping of red cells caused by the formation of antibody bridges between antigens on different cells

agglutinin . . . . an antibody causing agglutination

agglutinogen . . . . used in the Wiener theory of Rh to describe an antigen which is made up of parts or factors, each of which reacts with a specific antibody

AIHA . . . . autoimmune hemolytic anemia

albumin . . . . one of the three major plasma proteins — albumin, globulin, fibrinogen; *see* bovine albumin

allele . . . . any one of a series of genes which may occupy a given locus on each of a pair of homologous chromosomes

allelomorph . . . . now generally shortened to allele

allergic response . . . . a hypersensitive reaction to a particular substance; the target organs are usually the skin, the respiratory tract and the gastrointestinal tract

alloagglutinin . . . . an agglutinin from one individual that reacts with antigens of another individual of the same species

alpha-methyldopa . . . . a drug commonly used to treat high blood pressure

amino acid . . . . the building blocks of proteins; an organic acid carrying amino groups

amniocentesis . . . . transabdominal insertion of a needle into the amnionic sac to obtain amnionic fluid

amnionic fluid . . . . fluid within the amnionic sac surrounding the fetus

amorph . . . . a silent gene; a gene for which there is no known gene product

amphipathic . . . . of or relating to molecules with characteristically opposite properties, e.g., both hydrophilic and hydrophobic

anamnestic response . . . . the rapid reappearance of an antibody following exposure to an antigen to which the person has already developed a primary response

anaphylactic reaction . . . . an exaggerated allergic reaction to foreign proteins characterized by smooth muscle contraction and capillary dilatation resulting in gastrointestinal symptoms, hypotension and shock

antibody . . . . a substance present in the plasma, produced as a result of antigenic stimulation and capable of reacting with the specific antigen that caused its production

antibody screening test . . . . a test used to detect unexpected antibodies in serum

anticoagulant . . . . any substance that prevents coagulation of blood

antigen . . . . a substance capable of inducing the body to form antibodies; *see* blood group antigens

antiglobulin test . . . . *see* direct antiglobulin test and indirect antiglobulin test

anti-human serum . . . . anti-human globulin serum; a reagent usually made in rabbits immunized with purified human serum components

antipyretic . . . . an agent used to reduce fever

antiserum . . . . a reagent that contains an antibody or antibodies

aplastic anemia	a form of anemia characterized by a decrease in all the formed elements (cells) of peripheral blood
ascites	an accumulation of serous fluid in the abdominal cavity
autoantibody	an atypical antibody in the serum of an individual that agglutinates or sensitizes his own red blood cells
autoimmune hemolytic anemia	an acquired form of anemia in which an individual's antibodies (autoantibodies) destroy his own red blood cells; abbreviated AIHA
autologous	designating products or components of the same individual
autosome	any chromosome other than the sex chromosomes
B cells	the lymphocytes which, on stimulation by an antigen, differentiate into plasma cells that produce antibody
bilipid membrane (bilipid layer)	the membrane that forms the external structure of all cells and consists of a bilayer of phospholipids
bilirubin	the breakdown product resulting from the degradation of hemoglobin by the cells of the reticuloendothelial system
blood group antigens	antigens present on red blood cells
blood grouping	the process of testing red blood cells to determine which antigens are present and which are absent
blood grouping serum	reagent containing antibodies to blood group antigens
Bombay phenotype	a rare blood type occurring when no *H* gene is inherited
bovine albumin	a reagent consisting of a solution of albumin produced from the serum of cows
bursa	bursa of Fabricius; an organ in chickens which processes precursor lymphocytes into potential antibody-producing cells (B cells)
CAD	cold agglutinin disease; (a form of polyagglutination is called Cad)
chimera	an individual whose body contains two genetically different cell lines derived from two separate zygotes
chromosomes	structures within the cell nucleus that store and transmit genetic information
clone	a population of cells derived from a single cell by repeated mitosis
codon	genetic message unit made up of three adjacent nucleotides; each codon specifies a particular amino acid in a polypeptide
cold agglutinin disease	autoimmune hemolytic anemia caused by cold agglutinins; abbreviated CAD
cold antibody	an antibody that reacts optimally *in vitro* at temperatures below 20° to 25°C
compatibility test	commonly used as a synonym for crossmatch; more appropriately, all tests performed on donors and recipients to determine compatibility of blood
complement	a group of enzymatic proteins found in normal serum, some of which become associated with the cell membrane following interaction of antibody with its corresponding red cell antigen

complement fixation	the attachment of complement components to a cell following interaction of an antibody with its corresponding antigen
congenital hemolytic anemia . .	inherited hemolytic disorder; anemia, present at birth, in which the life span of the red blood cells is reduced
Coombs test	antiglobulin test; named for R.R. Coombs, who developed the test
crossing over	the interchange of segments of homologous chromosomes during meiosis, resulting in new combinations of genes
crossmatch	a test for incompatibility in which the serum of the recipient is tested with the red blood cells of each prospective donor
cytoplasm	the protoplasm of a cell exclusive of the nucleus
deoxyribonucleic acid	the nucleic acid that carries genetic information; abbreviated DNA
direct antiglobulin test	a test for the presence of antibody attached to red blood cells *in vivo*
DNA	deoxyribonucleic acid
Dolichos biflorus	anti-A_1 lectin; the plant from which seeds are harvested to prepare the lectin
dosage effect	the variation in quantity of an antigen on the red blood cells as a result of the expression of one gene or two like genes
double dose	the quantity of antigen produced by an individual homozygous for a particular gene
D (Rh_o)	the major Rh factor
edema	the presence of abnormal amounts of fluid in the intracellular tissue spaces of the body
en bloc	in a lump; as a whole (French)
epitope	a single antigenic determinant
erythrocyte	red blood cell
erythropoiesis	formation and development of red blood cells
expected antibodies	those antibodies regularly present in individuals who lack the reciprocal antigen, stimulated by exposure to naturally-occurring non-self antigens; anti-A and anti-B
extramedullary hemopoiesis . .	the formation and development of red blood cells outside the bone marrow
extravascular transfusion reaction	the response to transfusion of incompatible blood characterized by destruction of transfused red blood cells, primarily in the spleen
Fab piece	that fragment of the immunoglobulin molecule that has the ability to combine with antigen, consisting of portions of both heavy chains and all of both light chains; Fragment *a*ntigen *b*inding
factor	a term used to designate the part of an agglutinogen that reacts with antibody; antigenic determinant; epitope
Fc piece	that portion of the immunoglobulin molecule that does not combine with the antigen; it consists of portions of the two heavy chains; Fragment *c*rystallizable

febrile nonhemolytic reaction ... a transitory response characterized by fever, usually due to antibodies specific for the antigens of white blood cells and/or platelets

fibrinogen .... a major plasma protein that participates in coagulation, being converted to fibrin in the presence of thrombin

forward grouping .... red cell grouping; testing red blood cells for A and/or B antigens

fucosyl transferase .... an enzyme that catalyzes the transfer of fucose

gamma globulin .... serum protein that has antibody activity

gene cluster .... a set of contiguous genes inherited as a unit but which act individually

gene complex .... *see* gene cluster

genetic code .... the sequence of codons in a chromosome that governs transmission of genetic information

genome .... the complete set of hereditary factors contained in a haploid set of chromosomes

genotype .... the genetic constitution of an individual for a particular trait

globoside .... an oligosaccharide chain that forms the structure of the P antigen

globulin .... one of the major plasma proteins; can be divided into alpha globulin, beta globulin (complement) and gamma globulin (antibodies)

glucose-6-phosphate
dehydrogenase .... an enzyme of the pentose phosphate pathway which, when deficient, causes red blood cells to be more susceptible to oxidative denaturation; abbreviated G6PD

glycolipid .... a sugar-containing lipid derived from sphingosine; some glycolipids have only one sugar attached but those with blood group specificity have complex sugar chains attached

glycophorin A .... MN SGP; a sialoglycoprotein that protrudes from the red blood cell membrane and carries the antigenic determinants of M and N in the MNSs system

glycophorin B .... Ss SGP; a sialoglycoprotein that protrudes from the red blood cell membrane and carries the antigenic determinants of S and s in the MNSs system

glycoprotein .... a complex of one or more chains of sugar residues attached to a protein (polypeptide)

G6PD .... glucose-6-phosphate dehydrogenase

granulocyte .... any cell containing granules, especially a leukocyte containing neutrophilic, basophilic or eosinophilic granules in its cytoplasm

haptoglobin .... a glycoprotein which binds free hemoglobin

H chain .... heavy chain of immunoglobulin molecules; *see* type I H chain and type II H chain

HDN .... hemolytic disease of the newborn

hemoglobin .... the oxygen-carrying pigment of red blood cells

hemoglobinopathy .... a disease in which the structure of the protein moiety of hemoglobin is altered

hemoglobinuria	the presence of free hemoglobin in the urine
hemolysis	red blood cell destruction
hemolytic anemia	anemia caused by excessive *in vivo* destruction of red blood cells
hemolytic disease of the newborn	anemia of the newborn due to fetal red cell destruction by maternally-formed antibodies which have crossed the placenta; abbreviated HDN
hemosiderin	an insoluble form of iron; when it is produced in excess, as in chronically transfused patients, it accumulates in renal cells and other tissues
hemosiderinuria	the presence of free hemosiderin in the urine
hereditary elliptocytosis	a form of congenital hemolytic anemia resulting from abnormalities in the red blood cell membrane; the red cells are elliptical
hereditary spherocytosis	a form of congenital hemolytic anemia resulting from abnormalities in the red blood cell membrane; the red cells are spherical rather than biconcave
hereditary stomatocytosis	a form of congenital hemolytic anemia resulting from abnormalities in the red blood cell membranes; in fixed smears the center of the red cells appears to be "mouth-shaped"
heterogeneous	composed of dissimilar elements; not uniform
heterozygous	having two different alleles at the corresponding loci of the paired chromosomes
hinge region	the area of flexibility on the immunoglobulin molecule where the L chain attaches to the H chain
homozygous	having identical alleles at the corresponding loci of the paired chromosomes
H substance	a soluble blood group substance; soluble H antigen
hybridoma	myeloma cells fused with antibody-producing spleen cells; they can be cloned by growing on culture media and used to produce antibody
hydrophilic	having an affinity for water
hydrophobic	antagonistic to water
hydrops fetalis	a severe form of HDN in which the infant has generalized edema, severe anemia and congestive heart failure — usually stillborn
hyperbilirubinemia	excessive concentration of bilirubin in the blood
hypogammaglobulinemia	abnormally low levels of gamma globulin in the blood
hypoproteinemia	abnormally low levels of protein in the blood
idiopathic	of unknown cause
IgG	immunoglobulin G
IgM	immunoglobulin M
immune hemolytic anemia	an acquired condition in which anemia is caused by immune destruction of red blood cells
immune response	reaction of the body following exposure to an antigen; *see* primary response and secondary response

immunogen	an antigen that stimulates antibody production
immunogenicity	antigenicity; the ability of an antigen to stimulate production of its corresponding antibody in an individual who lacks the antigen
immunoglobulin	a protein (globulin) with antibody activity
incomplete antibodies	antibodies that sensitize cells but do not agglutinate them without the addition of potentiators or anti-human globulin serum
indirect antiglobulin test	a test for antibody that was attached to red blood cells *in vitro*
inflammatory response	a localized protective response to injury or destruction of tissues which serves to destroy, dilute or wall off the injurious agent and the injured tissue
inhibitor	the product of a gene that inhibits the expression of another gene
intravascular transfusion reaction	the response to transfusion of incompatible blood characterized by hemolysis of transfused cells in the bloodstream resulting in a rapid, severe clinical response; the cell destruction is mediated by the action of antigen, antibody and complement
in vitro	"in glass"; occurring outside the body
in vivo	occurring in the body
ischemia	local deficiency in the blood supply; localized tissue anemia
kernicterus	bilirubin pigmentation of the central nervous system — especially basal ganglia — accompanied by degeneration of nerve cells
lectins	a group of naturally-occurring materials (usually from plant sources) that react specifically with blood group antigens
leukemia	a malignant disease of the blood-forming organs in which there is distorted development and proliferation of leukocytes
low ionic strength solutions ...	solutions in which the concentrations of Na^+ and Cl^- are lower than in normal saline
lymphocyte	a mononuclear leukocyte which plays a major role in the immune response
lymphoma	a general term for any neoplastic disorder of the lymphoid tissue, including Hodgkin's disease
lysis	destruction of cells
macrophage	a phagocytic cell of the reticuloendothelial system
major crossmatch	test for incompatibility between patient serum and donor cells
messenger RNA	a single-stranded ribonucleic acid that transmits information from DNA in the nucleus to the protein-forming system of the cytoplasm; abbreviated mRNA
minor crossmatch	a test for incompatibility between patient cells and donor serum
minus-minus phenotype	null phenotype
mixed-field agglutination	a reaction in which some of the red cells are clumped while many cells remain unagglutinated
modifier gene	used alternatively with regulator gene in this text

monoclonal antibodies	antibodies produced by a clone of cells derived from a single cell and therefore identical to each other in specificity, immunoglobulin class and all other properties inherent in the original antibody-producing cell
monocyte	a large mononuclear phagocytic leukocyte
mRNA	messenger ribonucleic acid
mutation	a heritable change (addition, loss or rearrangement) of genetic material
myeloma	a tumor made up of cells of the type normally found in the bone marrow
naturally-occurring antibody . .	a term widely used to describe antibodies produced in response to non-erythrocyte antigens
neutralizing substances	blood group substances that neutralize their corresponding antibodies in human sera; soluble antigens; *see* substance
nucleotides	the building blocks of DNA and RNA; composed of a phosphate group attached to a nucleoside; the nucleoside is a purine or pyrimidine base to which a sugar is attached — ribose in RNA and deoxyribose in DNA
null phenotype	a phenotype in which there is little, if any, antigen detectable on the red cells; minus-minus phenotype
oligosaccharide	a carbohydrate consisting of disaccharides, bisaccharides and tetrasaccharides; when hydrolyzed they yield a small number of monosaccharides
para-Bombay phenotype	phenotype describing individuals who lack H chains on their red cells but have H substance in secretions
paragloboside	an oligosaccharide that serves as the substrate for the transferase that produces the P_1 antigen
peptide bond	the bond formed between the carboxyl group of one amino acid and the amino group of another in a polypeptide chain
phagocyte	any cell that can engulf microorganisms, foreign particles or certain other cells
phenotype	the visible expression of a genotype; the physiological, biochemical and physical make-up of an individual as described by observation and test results
phospholipid	a compound comprising the major form of lipid in cell membranes; it is composed of glycerol, fatty acids, a phosphate group and a nitrogenous group
physiological jaundice	a relatively mild, non-hemolytic jaundice due to unconjugated bilirubin
PK	pyruvate kinase
plasma	the fluid portion of the blood in which the formed elements (cells) are suspended
plasma cells	the cells that develop from B cells on stimulation by an antigen and which produce antibodies

polyagglutination . . . .   agglutination by a number of sera (or specific lectins) due to exposure of normally hidden antigens which form part of the red cell membrane; most adult sera contain antibodies to these normally hidden antigens

polymorphic . . . .   existing in multiple forms; describing a system in which several phenotypes are commonly found

polypeptide chain . . . .   a chain of amino acids joined by peptide bonds

polyvinylpyrrolidone . . . .   a synthetic potentiator that promotes agglutination; abbreviated PVP

potentiator . . . .   an additive incorporated into a test system; it is designed to enhance the rate of antibody uptake by a specific antigen or the strength of visible agglutination

precursor chain . . . .   an oligosaccharide that is the substrate for the action of one or more transferases

primary response . . . .   antibody production in response to the first exposure to a foreign immunogen

proteolytic enzymes . . . .   enzymes that catalyze the breaking of certain peptide bonds in proteins

PVP . . . .   polyvinylpyrrolidone

pyruvate kinase . . . .   the enzyme that catalyzes the ATP-ADP reaction; deficiency alters the energy metabolism of red blood cells and may cause hemolytic episodes; abbreviated PK

reagent red cells . . . .   red blood cells of known antigen make-up which are used in testing for the presence of antibodies

red cell grouping . . . .   testing red cells for blood group antigens — often specifically a test used to determine the ABO group

regulator genes . . . .   genes whose products control the rate at which the products of other genes are synthesized

RES . . . .   reticuloendothelial system

reticuloendothelial system . . . .   a functional rather than anatomical system of cells whose primary function is phagocytosis; the cells involved are the monocytes of peripheral blood and the fixed macrophages of the liver, spleen, bone marrow, lymph nodes, lungs, connective tissue, and brain; abbreviated RES

reverse grouping . . . .   a test used to determine ABO group in which the individual's serum is tested for the presence of expected anti-A and/or anti-B using known group A and group B cells

Rh immune globulin . . . .   a sterile solution derived from human plasma containing anti-D (anti-Rh_o), used to suppress an immune response to D (Rh_o) antigen

Rh negative . . . .   a blood type characterized by the absence of D (Rh_o) antigen and its variant D^u from the red blood cells

Rh positive . . . .   a blood type characterized by the presence of D (Rh_o) antigen or its variant D^u on the red blood cells

ribosomes . . . .   structures in the cytoplasm of the cell that are the sites of protein synthesis

RNA	ribonucleic acid
secondary response	the rapid reappearance of antibody in the blood following exposure to an antigen to which a subject had previously developed a primary response
secretor	an individual whose secretions (especially saliva) contain water-soluble A, B or H substances, depending on the ABO blood group
secretor genes	the genes (*Se* and *se*) that control secretion of A, B and H substances into saliva and other body fluids
self-recognition	the process by which the body identifies its own constituents, thus precluding the immune response to autologous antigens
sensibilization	the state of immunization in which no antibodies can be detected
sensitization	the initial exposure of an individual to a specific antigen resulting in an immune response
sensitized cells	red blood cells that have incomplete antibodies attached to the antigens of their surfaces
sensitizing antibodies	incomplete antibodies
sequester	to detach or separate a portion from the whole; e.g., separation of certain red blood cells from the blood by the spleen
serum	the clear liquid remaining after blood clots; it contains no cells or fibrinogen
serum grouping	reverse grouping
sex chromosomes	chromosomes that are associated with determination of sex; designated X and Y
SGP	sialoglycoprotein
sialoglycoprotein	a glycoprotein in which the sugar is primarily sialic acid; abbreviated SGP
sickle-cell anemia	a hereditary form of hemolytic anemia due to abnormal hemoglobin and characterized by red blood cells which become sickle-shaped under conditions of reduced oxygen tension
silent gene	amorph; a gene for which there does not appear to be any product
single dose	the quantity of antigen produced by an individual heterozygous for a particular gene
SLE	systemic lupus erythematosus
slipping plane	*see* surface of shear
specificity	the characteristic of an antibody to react exclusively with one antigen and no other
stroma	the supporting tissues or matrix of an organ or certain cells, as in the part of the red blood cell remaining after the hemoglobin has been removed
structural genes	the genes that direct the construction of proteins
substance	in immunohematology, an antigen in solution
substrate	a receptor for the action of an enzyme

surface of shear	the edge of the ion cloud surrounding a red blood cell; the surface at which the positive and negative ions are in equilibrium; it functions as the effective surface of the cell in relation to the approach of another cell
systemic lupus erythematosus	a disorder of the connective tissues involving abnormal immunological responses and characterized by inflammatory skin eruptions; abbreviated SLE
T cells	lymphocytes processed by the thymus gland, responsible for cell-mediated immunity; they interact with B cells either to aid or to suppress antibody production in the presence of antigen
thymocytes	T cell precursors during their processing by the thymus
thymus	the lymphoid organ necessary for the development and maturation of immunological defense; it processes lymphocytes into T cells
transferase	an enzyme that catalyzes the transfer of a chemical group from one molecule (donor) to another (substrate)
transfusion reaction	any adverse reaction to the transfusion of whole blood or blood components
transudation	the passage of serum or other body fluid through a membrane
type I H chain	the type of H chain predominant in body fluids
type II H chain	the type of H chain that forms an integral part of the red blood cell membrane
unexpected antibodies	antibodies other than anti-A and anti-B; antibodies found in the sera of a small number of individuals, caused by exposure to red blood cells carrying antigens unlike their own
urobilinogen	a colorless compound formed in the intestines by reduction of conjugated bilirubin
warm antibody	an antibody that reacts optimally at 37°C
zeta potential	the electrostatic potential measured between the red cell membrane and the slipping plane of the same cell
zygote	the diploid cell formed by the fusion of sperm and ovum

Index

Sources of Additional Information

Bellanti JA: *Immunology II*. Philadelphia, WB Saunders Company, 1978.

Blood Group Antigens & Antibodies as Applied to Hemolytic Disease of the Newborn. Raritan, NJ, Ortho Diagnostic Systems Inc., 1968.

Gardner EJ, Snustad DP: *Principles of Genetics*, ed 6. New York, John Wiley & Sons, Inc., 1981.

Keeton WT: *Biological Science*, ed 3. New York, WW Norton & Company, Inc., 1980.

Mollison PL: *Blood Transfusion in Clinical Medicine*, ed 6. Oxford, Blackwell Scientific Publications, 1979.

Petz LD, Garratty G: *Acquired Immune Hemolytic Anemias*. New York, Churchill Livingstone, 1980.

Petz LD, Swisher SN (eds): *Clinical Practice of Blood Transfusion*. New York, Churchill Livingstone, 1981.

Race RR, Sanger R: *Blood Groups in Man*, ed 6. Oxford, Blackwell Scientific Publications, 1975.

Roitt IM: *Essential Immunology*, ed 4. Oxford, Blackwell Scientific Publications, 1980.

Sandler SG, Nusbacher J, Schanfield MS (eds): *Immunobiology of the Erythrocyte*. New York, Alan R. Liss, Inc., 1980.

Stryer L: *Biochemistry*, ed 2. San Francisco, WH Freeman & Company, 1981.

Technical Manual, ed 8. Washington, DC, American Association of Blood Banks, 1981.

Watson JD: *Molecular Biology of the Gene*, ed 3. Menlo Park, CA, The Benjamin-Cummings Publishing Company, 1976.

Weissman IL, Hood LE, Wood WB: *Essential Concepts in Immunology*. Menlo Park, CA, The Benjamin-Cummings Publishing Company, 1978.